Transoesophageal Echocardiography

Transoesophageal echocardiography (TOE/TEE) in cardiac patients is now almost routine. Its use in cardiac monitoring has also extended to include critically ill patients for non-cardiac surgery and the intensive care setting. Specific accreditation is required prior to practice of TOE/TEE involving a written examination and a documented logbook of experience. This book has been specifically designed to help candidates pass the written exam and has been structured around the syllabus. Providing a summary of all relevant information, this is an invaluable study aid. Lists of further reading material are provided with every topic, including guidelines and safety, cardiomyopathies, heart disease, haemodynamic calculations and many more. Each chapter ends with a series of exam-style questions for self-assessment. An extremely useful book for trainee anaesthetists, intensivists, trainee cardiologists and cardiac surgeons.

Andrew Roscoe is a consultant in cardiothoracic anaesthesia at Wythenshawe Hospital in Manchester, UK.

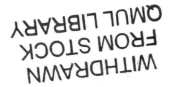

Transoesophageal Echocardiography

Study Guide and Practice Questions

Dr Andrew Roscoe, F.R.C.A

Consultant in Cardiothoracic Anaesthesia
Wythenshawe Hospital, Manchester, UK

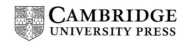

CAMBRIDGE UNIVERSITY PRESS

CAMBRIDGE UNIVERSITY PRESS
Cambridge, New York, Melbourne, Madrid, Cape Town, Singapore, São Paulo

Cambridge University Press
The Edinburgh Building, Cambridge CB2 8RU, UK

Published in the United States of America by Cambridge University Press, New York

www.cambridge.org
Information on this title: www.cambridge.org/9780521689601

First published 2007

Printed in the United Kingdom at the University Press, Cambridge

A catalog record for this publication is available from the British Library

ISBN-13 978-0-521-68960-1 paperback

Contents

List of abbreviations

A	amplitude
AC	attenuation coefficient
AF	atrial fibrillation
AI	aortic incompetence
A/L	antero-lateral
AMVL	anterior mitral valve leaflet
AS	aortic stenosis
ASD	atrial septal defect
AV	aortic valve
A-V	atrio-ventricular
AVA	aortic valve area
AVC	aortic valve closes
AVN	atrio-ventricular node
AVO	aortic valve opens
BP	blood pressure
BSA	body surface area
BUR	beam uniformity ratio
CC	costal cartilage
CCF	congestive cardiac failure
CFD	colour flow Doppler
Cn	compliance
CO	cardiac output
CPB	cardiopulmonary bypass
CS	coronary sinus
CW	continuous wave
CWD	continuous wave Doppler
DBP	diastolic blood pressure
depT	depressurization time

DF	duty factor
DT	deceleration time
EF	ejection fraction
ERO	effective regurgitant orifice
ET	ejection time
f_D	Doppler frequency
FD	focal depth
FO	foramen ovale
FS	fractional shortening
HOCM	hypertrophic obstructive cardiomyopathy
HV	hepatic vein
HVLT	half value layer thickness
I	intensity
IAS	interatrial septum
ICU	intensive care unit
IHD	ischaemic heart disease
IPP	intrapericardial pressure
IRC	intensity reflection coefficient
ITC	intensity transmitted coefficient
IVC	inferior vena cava
IVRT	isovolumic relaxation time
IVS	interventricular septum
LA	left atrium
LAA	left atrial appendage
LAD	left anterior descending coronary artery
LAP	left atrial pressure
LARRD	longitudinal resolution
LATA	lateral resolution
LAX	long axis view
LBBB	left bundle branch block
LCA	left coronary artery
LCC	left coronary cusp
LCCA	left common carotid artery
LCx	left circumflex coronary artery
LGC	lateral gain compensation

LLPV	left lower pulmonary vein
LPA	left pulmonary artery
LSCA	left subclavian artery
LSE	left sternal edge
LUPV	left upper pulmonary vein
LV	left ventricle
LVEDP	left ventricular end diastolic pressure
LVEDV	left ventricular end diastolic volume
LVESV	left ventricular end systolic volume
LVH	left ventricular hypertrophy
LVIDd	left ventricular internal diameter in diastole
LVIDs	left ventricular internal diameter in systole
LVM	left ventricular mass
LVOT	left ventricular outflow tract
LVP	left ventricular pressure
LVSP	left ventricular systolic pressure
MAPSE	mitral annular plane systolic excursion
MG	mean gradient
MI	myocardial infarction
MM	motion mode
MR	mitral regurgitation
MRI	magnetic resonance imaging
MV	mitral valve
MVA	mitral valve area
MVC	mitral valve closes
MVL	mitral valve leaflet
MVO	mitral valve opens
NCC	non-coronary cusp
P	power
PA	pulmonary artery
PADP	pulmonary artery diastolic pressure
PAP	pulmonary artery pressure
PD	pulse duration
PDA	patent ductus arteriosus
PE	pulmonary embolism

P/E	piezo-electric
PFO	patent foramen ovale
PG	pressure gradient
PHT	pressure half-time
PI	pulmonary incompetence
PISA	proximal isovelocity area
PM	papillary muscle
P/M	postero-medial
PMVL	posterior mitral valve leaflet
PRF	pulse repetition frequency
PRP	pulse repetition period
PS	pulmonary stenosis
PV	pulmonary valve
PVs	pulmonary veins
PW	pulse wave
PWD	pulse wave Doppler
PZT-5	lead zirconate titanate – 5
RA	right atrium
RAP	right atrial pressure
RBBB	right bundle branch block
rbc	red blood cell
RCA	right coronary artery
RCC	right coronary cusp
RF	regurgitant fraction
RLN	recurrent laryngeal nerve
RLPV	right lower pulmonary vein
RPA	right pulmonary artery
RSE	right sternal edge
RUPV	right upper pulmonary vein
RV	right ventricle
RVH	right ventricular hypertrophy
RVOT	right ventricular outflow tract
RVP	right ventricular pressure
RVSP	right ventricular systolic pressure
RWMA	regional wall motion abnormality

SAM	systolic anterior motion
SAN	sino-atrial node
SAPA	spatial average, pulse average
SATA	spatial average, temporal average
SATP	spatial average, temporal peak
SAX	short axis view
SBP	systolic blood pressure
SCA	sickle cell anaemia
SLE	systemic lupus erythematosus
SPL	spatial pulse length
SPPA	spatial peak, pulse average
SPTA	spatial peak, temporal average
SPTP	spatial peak, temporal peak
STJ	sino-tubular junction
SV	stroke volume
SVI	stroke volume index
SVR	systemic vascular resistance
TA	truncus arteriosus
TAA	thoracic aortic aneurysm
TAPSE	tricuspid annular plane systolic excursion
TAPVD	total anomalous pulmonary venous drainage
TB	tuberculosis
T_d	time delay
TDI	tissue Doppler imaging
TGA	transposition of great arteries
TGC	time gain compensation
TMF	transmitral flow
TOE	transoesophageal echocardiography
TR	tricuspid regurgitation
TS	tricuspid stenosis
TTE	transthoracic echocardiography
TTF	transtricuspid flow
TV	tricuspid valve
TVA	tricuspid valve area
TVC	tricuspid valve closes

TVL	tricuspid valve leaflet
TVO	tricuspid valve opens
TX	transducer
U/S	ultrasound
Vcf	velocity of circumferential fibre shortening
VSD	ventricular septal defect
VTI	velocity–time integral
WPW	Wolfe–Parkinson–White syndrome
Z	impedance

Foreword

Over the past decade there has been a dramatic increase in the use of transoesophageal echocardiography (TOE) in the perioperative setting among all disciplines caring for the cardiac patient. Where TOE used to be used mainly by cardiologists in the echocardiography laboratory, we now recognize its value in the operating theatre, cardiac catheter laboratory, and intensive care unit. TOE has become the gold standard perioperative cardiac monitor and diagnostic tool for certain cardiac surgical procedures. Its role has also been extended to critically ill or unstable patients for non-cardiac procedures and the general intensive care arena. The increasing involvement of anaesthetists and of other specialities at an advanced level has promoted the team approach to perioperative patient care. The rapid advances in the use of this technology have also resulted in a critical need for interdisciplinary training.

The development of training and certification in echocardiography has been a long and intensive process in Europe and the USA. Excellent comprehensive TOE courses have been available and working groups on TOE have published extensive practice and training guidelines on both sides of the Atlantic and in Japan. The American Society of Cardiovascular Anesthesiologists (SCA) developed the first formal examination in perioperative TOE in 1998. The SCA and the American Society of Echocardiography (ASE) then combined forces to establish the National Board of Echocardiography (NBE), which had the responsibility to further administer examinations and develop a certification process in clinical echocardiography. Europe followed a similar route with the Association of Cardiothoracic Anaesthetists (ACTA) joining forces with the British Society of Echocardiography

(BSE) to establish an accreditation process in TOE with its first examination held in the UK in 2003. Since then the European Association of Cardiothoracic Anaesthesiologists (EACTA) and the European Society of Echocardiography (ESE) produced its own European TOE examination and accreditation process in 2005. In 2004, the Japanese Society of Cardiovascular Anesthesiologists launched their first TOE competency examination.

The purpose of these accreditation processes is to enable recognition of special competence in perioperative echocardiography against an objective standard, and all of them consist of two parts. With the *practical part*, the candidate must demonstrate adequate training and competency through a supervised residency program or logbook. The *theoretical part* requires the successful completion of a multiple choice and image clip examination.

With his experience in learning, practicing and teaching perioperative echocardiography in North America and in the UK, the author fills a certain niche with this book. It is not intended to be a comprehensive reference book. In contrast to the vast amount of information on echocardiography already available both in print and online, this book provides the aspiring echocardiographer with a valuable summarized resource to prepare for any of the perioperative echocardiography examinations. It gives any examination candidate a convenient framework onto which further knowledge can be added. Both the American and the European perioperative TOE examination syllabus is well covered in a concise manner. The *Perioperative Transoesophageal Echocardiography Exam Notes* contains all the critical physics equations, standard values and plenty of diagrams in a highly absorbable way. Each chapter also concludes with a series of exam-style self-assessment questions to emphasize important facts and practice for the exam.

Cardiac surgery and anaesthesia have come a long way since the late 1970s when TOE was introduced into the perioperative arena. The development of many surgical procedures and the reduction in perioperative morbidity and mortality can be directly related to the use of TOE. There rests a great responsibility on any clinician performing a diagnostic perioperative TOE. This book will certainly contribute not only to help preparation for the examinations, but also to raise the standard of our practice and patient care.

Steve Konstadt
Justiaan Swanevelder

Physics of ultrasound

Basic principles

Nature of ultrasound

Sound = longitudinal, mechanical wave
  particles move parallel to direction of travel

Audible sound < 20 kHz
Ultrasound > 20 kHz
Sound cannot travel through a vacuum

Four acoustic variables

  Density (g/l)
  Pressure (kPa)
  Temperature (K)
  Particle motion (m)

Compressions: high density/pressure/temperature/motion +
Rarefactions: low density/pressure/temperature/motion
(Fig. 1.1)
Transthoracic echo (TTE) ~ 2–5 MHz
Transoesophageal echo (TOE) ~ 3.5–7 MHz

Sound is described by
  Propagation speed (m/s)
  Frequency (Hz)
  Wavelength (m)

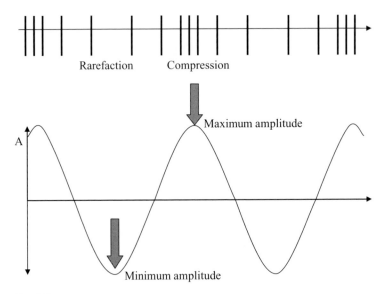

Rarefaction   Compression

Maximum amplitude

A

Minimum amplitude

Fig. 1.1

Period (s)
Amplitude (kPa, g/l, K, m, dB)
Power (W)
Intensity (W/cm^2)

Propagation speed (*v* or *c*)

c = speed of sound   Units = m/s or mm/µs
Determined by the medium through which the wave travels
Soft tissue (heart) = 1540 m/s = 1.54 mm/µs
Speed affected by density and stiffness of medium
↑density → ↓speed
↑stiffness (= bulk modulus) → ↑speed
Elasticity and compressibility = opposite to stiffness
↑elasticity/compressibility → ↓speed
All sound travels through a specific medium at the same speed
(Table 1.1)

Table 1.1 Speed of sound in different media

Tissue	Speed of sound (m/s)
Air	331
Lung	500
Fat	1450
Brain	1541
Liver	1549
Muscle	1585
Bone	>3000

Frequency (f)

f = number of cycles per second   Units = Hz

U/S > 20 kHz

Determined by sound source

Affects penetration and axial resolution

Period (T)

T = length of time to complete one cycle   Units = s

U/S = 0.1–0.5 µs

Determined by sound source

Reciprocal of frequency $T = 1/f$

Wavelength (λ)

λ = distance occupied by a single cycle   Units = m

U/S = 0.1–0.8 mm

Determined by sound source and medium

λ influences axial resolution

Velocity (v), frequency (f) and wavelength (λ) associated by the equation

$$v = f\lambda$$

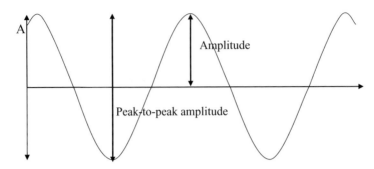

Fig. 1.2

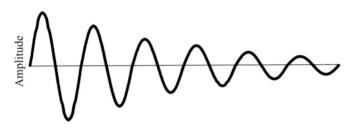

Fig. 1.3

Amplitude (*A*)

A = max. variation in acoustic variable   Units = kPa, g/l, K, m, dB,
   i.e. difference between <u>mean</u> and <u>max.</u> values
(Fig. 1.2)

Decibel (dB) = logarithmic relative unit of measure of A
   i.e. difference between two values
      e.g. ↑ by 30 dB = ↑A by 10 × 10 × 10 (×1000)

Determined by sound source
Changed by sonographer
Amplitude decreases as sound wave travels = **attenuation**
(Fig. 1.3)

Power (*P*)

P = rate of work/rate of energy transfer   Units = W

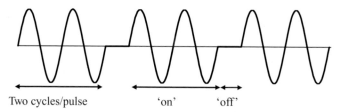

Two cycles/pulse   'on'   'off'

Fig. 1.4

Determined by sound source
Changed by sonographer

$$P = A^2$$

Intensity (I)

I = concentration of energy/power in a sound beam
Units = W/cm^2
Determined by sound source
Changed by sonographer
U/S $I = 0.1–100 \ mW/cm^2$

$$I = P/area$$

Pulsed ultrasound

Pulse = collection of cycles travelling together
    individual 'cycles' make up the 'pulse'
    'pulse' moves as one
    'pulse' has beginning and end
Two components:
    'cycle' or 'on' time
    'receive' or 'off' or 'dead' time (Fig. 1.4)
Pulsed U/S described by:
    pulse duration (PD)
    pulse repetition frequency (PRF)
    pulse repetition period (PRP)

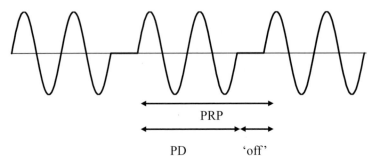

PRP

PD   'off'

Fig. 1.5

   spatial pulse length (SPL)
   duty factor (DF)

Pulse duration (PD)

PD = time from start of one pulse to end of pulse   Units $=$ s
    = 'on' time (Fig. 1.5)
Determined by:
   number of cycles in a pulse ('ringing')
   period of each cycle
Characteristic of transducer/not changed by sonographer
TOE   PD $= 0.5$–3 μs

$$PD = \text{number of cycles} \times T \quad PD = \text{number of cycles}/f$$

Pulse repetition frequency (PRF)

PRF $=$ number of pulses per second   Units $=$ Hz
(Number of cycles per pulse *not* relevant)
Determined by sound source
Changed by sonographer by changing image depth

As image depth increases $\rightarrow$ PRF$\downarrow$
Sonographer $\uparrow$'dead' time by $\uparrow$image depth $= \downarrow$PRF
TOE   PRF $= 1$–10 kHz

$$PRF(kHz) = 75/\text{depth (cm)}$$

Pulse repetition period (PRP)

PRP = time from start of one pulse to start of next pulse

Units = s

PRP = 'on' time (PD) + 'off' time (Fig. 1.5)

Changed by sonographer by changing 'off' time

TOE   PRP = 0.1–1 ms

$$PRP \ (\mu s) = 13 \times depth \ (cm)$$

Spatial pulse length (SPL)

SPL = length in distance occupied by one pulse   Units = m

Determined by sound source and medium

Cannot be changed by sonographer

TOE   SPL = 0.1–1 mm

Determines axial resolution

i.e. short SPL → better axial resolution

$$SPL = number \ of \ cycles \times \lambda$$

Duty factor (DF)

DF = percentage of 'on' time compared to PRP   Units = %

Changed by sonographer by changing 'off' time

TOE   DF = 0.1–1% (i.e. lots of 'off'/listening time)

$$DF = PD/PRP$$

↑DF by:

   ↑PRF (more pulses/s)

   ↑PD (by changing transducer)

↓DF by:

   ↑PRP (by ↑'off' time)

   ↑image depth

DF = 100% = continuous wave (CW) U/S

DF = 0% = machine off

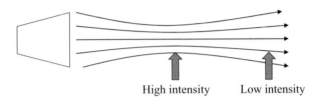

High intensity   Low intensity

Fig. 1.6

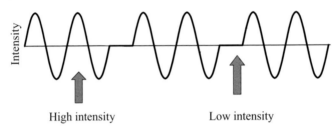

High intensity   Low intensity

Fig. 1.7

Properties of ultrasound

Intensity (*I*)

Described by:

(1) Spatial – U/S beam has different *I* at different locations (Fig. 1.6)
   Peak *I* = spatial peak (SP)
   Average *I* = spatial average (SA)
(2) Temporal – U/S beam has different *I* at different points in time
   (Fig. 1.7)
   Peak *I* = temporal peak (TP), i.e. 'on' time
   Average *I* = temporal average (TA), i.e. average of 'on' and 'off'
   For CW: TP = TA
(3) Pulse – U/S beam has average *I* for duration of pulse ('on')
   = pulse average (PA)

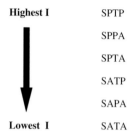

Highest I	SPTP
	SPPA
	SPTA
	SATP
	SAPA
Lowest I	SATA

SPTA relevant to tissue heating
For CW: SPTP = SPTA and SATP = SATA
When PW and CW have same SPTP/SATP
   CW has higher SPTA/SATA
PA > TA for PW

Beam uniformity ratio (BUR)
BUR = SP/SA factor
No units
Scale 1– ∞ (infinity)
Describes the spread of sound beam in space
TOE   BUR = 5–50

Attenuation
Decrease in A/P/I as sound wave travels (Fig. 1.3)
Units = −dB
In soft tissue: ↑f → ↑attenuation
Three components:
(1) absorption:
   energy transferred to cell in tissue by conversion to other form of energy
   sound → heat/vibration
(2) reflection:
   energy returned to source when it strikes a boundary between two media

(i) Specular reflections

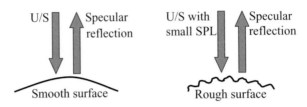

(ii) Scatter

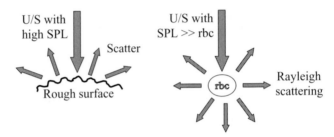

Fig. 1.8

(3) scatter:
 sound beam hits rough surface → sound wave redirected in several
 directions

Rayleigh scattering = when reflector << SPL (e.g. red blood cells)
 → scattering equal in all directions
(Fig. 1.8)
Attenuation coefficient (AC)
Units = −dB/cm
In soft tissue: ↑f→ ↑AC

$$AC = 0.5 \times f \text{ (MHz)}$$

Total attenuation = AC × path length (cm)
 ↑AC in: bone (absorption and reflection)
 air/lung (scatter)

Table 1.2 Effect of transducer frequency on attenuation coefficient (AC) and half-value layer thickness (HVLT)

Transducer f (MHz)	AC ($-dB/cm$)	HVLT (cm)
2	1	3
3	1.5	2
4	2	1.5
5	2.5	1.2
6	3	1

Half value layer thickness (HVLT)

HVLT = depth at which I falls by $\frac{1}{2} = -3$ dB Units = cm
(also called penetration depth and half boundary layer)
TOE HVLT = 0.25–2 cm (Table 1.2)
  HVLT = 3/AC HVLT = 6/f

Impedance (Z)

Z = resistance to sound propagation Units = Rayls
Calculated/not measured
Soft tissue = 1.25–1.75 MRayls
Reflection depends upon change in Z between two media
(Fig. 1.9)

$$Z = \rho \times v \text{ (density} \times \text{velocity)}$$

Intensity reflection coefficient (IRC)

IRC (%) = reflected I/incident I

Intensity transmitted coefficient (ITC)

ITC (%) = transmitted I/incident I
Clinically: Soft tissue IRC = 1% ITC = 99%
  Bone IRC = 99% ITC = 1%

With a 90° incident angle, reflection only occurs if $Z_1 \neq Z_2$
Greater the difference between Z_1 and $Z_2 \rightarrow \uparrow$IRC

$$\text{IRC (\%)} = [(Z_2 - Z_1)/(Z_2 + Z_1)]^2$$

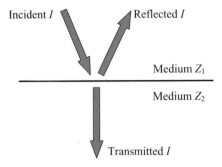

Incident I = transmitted I + reflected I

Fig. 1.9

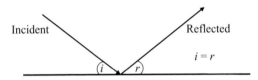

Fig. 1.10

With an oblique angle of incidence → reflection and refraction
Reflection: incident angle = reflected angle (Fig. 1.10)
Refraction: obeys Snell's Law (Fig. 1.11)
Velocity of transmitted beam > incident beam if $t > i$

Range

= time taken for pulse to travel from transducer to reflector and back
to transducer
= 'go–return' time

Distance to boundary (mm) = v (mm/μs) × range (μs)/2

$D = 1.54 \times \text{range}/2$

$D = 0.77 \times \text{range}$

13 μs rule: range = 13 μs → reflector depth = 10 mm
= 26 μs →   = 20 mm
= 39 μs →   = 30 mm

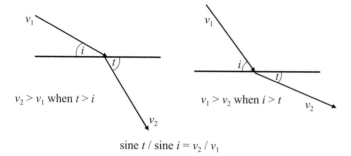

$v_2 > v_1$ when $t > i$

$v_1 > v_2$ when $i > t$

sine t / sine $i = v_2 / v_1$

Fig. 1.11

Transducers

Basic principles

Transducer (TX) = converts energy from one form to another
  acoustic → kinetic → electrical → heat

Piezoelectric (P/E) effect
= ability of a material to create a voltage
  when mechanically deformed
Reverse P/E effect = material changes shape when voltage applied
P/E materials = ferroelectric

Natural P/E materials
= quartz, Rochelle salts, tourmaline
Synthetic = Ba titanate, Pb titanate, Pb zirconate titanate (PZT)
U/S imagers – PZT-5 (also called 'ceramic')

Curie temperature
= temperature above which the P/E material
   loses its P/E effect because it depolarizes

Therefore: TX cannot be heated/sterilized/autoclaved

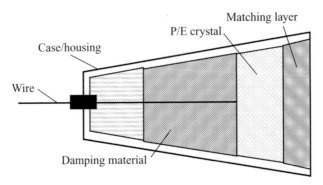

Fig. 1.12

Ultrasound transducers (Fig. 1.12) composed of:

(1)   active element: P/E crystal (PZT-5)
(2)   case:
      protects internal components
      insulates patient from electrical currents
(3)   wire:
      provides electrical contact with P/E crystal
      voltage from U/S system $\rightarrow$ vibration $\rightarrow$ U/S wave
      reception of signal $\rightarrow$ vibration $\rightarrow$ voltage to wire
(4)   matching layer:
      has impedance (Z) in-between that of TX and skin to prevent large
        reflection at skin
      Z of TX $\approx$ 33 MRayls
      Z of skin $\approx$ 1.5 MRayls
      $\rightarrow$ 96% IRC at skin
      Z of matching layer $\approx$ 7 MRayls
      Thickness of matching layer $= \lambda/4$
      Improves axial resolution
(5)   damping element:
      material bonded to active element
      epoxy resin impregnated with tungsten limits 'ringing'
      Improves axial resolution

'Ringing'

= P/E crystals have prolonged response to excitation
    → ↑PD → reduced axial resolution

Length of 'ringing' response = 'ringdown'
= number of half cycles required for oscillations of P/E crystal to decay
    to 10% (−20 dB) of the max peak-to-peak amplitude

Damping → ↓ringdown
        → absorbs U/S emitted from back face of TX, which causes
        interference by reflecting within housing of TX

Transducer frequencies

Resonant f of TX depends on thickness of P/E crystal
Max resonance occurs when thickness = $\lambda/2$

CW U/S: U/S f determined by and equal to f of voltage applied to P/E
    crystal
PW U/S: PRF determined by number of electrical pulses the machine
    delivers to P/E crystal

f of U/S determined by:
    thickness ($\lambda/2$)
    c in P/E crystal ($\sim$ 4–6 mm/μs)

$$f\ (\text{MHz}) = c\ (\text{mm}/\mu\text{s})/2 \times \text{thickness (mm)}$$

Sound beams

Beam diameter:
    starts same size as TX
    converges to focus
    diverges away from focus

Focus = location at minimum diameter (Fig. 1.13)
Focal depth (FD) = distance from TX to focus

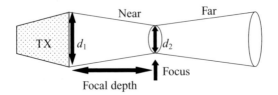

Near zone = Fresnel zone   At focus: $d_2 = d_1/2$
Far zone = Fraunhofer zone

Fig. 1.13

↑TX diameter → ↑FD/↓divergence

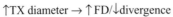

↓TX diameter → ↓FD/↑divergence

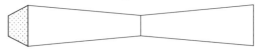

Fig. 1.14

Focal depth determined by:
   TX diameter
   f of U/S

$$FD = TX\ diam^2 \times f/6$$

Sound beam divergence
↑TX diameter → ↑FD/↓divergence
↓TX diameter → ↓FD/↑divergence (Fig. 1.14)

Focusing
= changing FD
↓FD → ↓diameter of beam
Lateral resolution improved by focusing

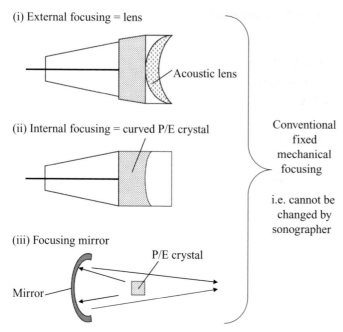

(i) External focusing = lens

Acoustic lens

(ii) Internal focusing = curved P/E crystal

(iii) Focusing mirror

P/E crystal

Mirror

Conventional
fixed
mechanical
focusing

i.e. cannot be
changed by
sonographer

Fig. 1.15

Types of focusing: (Fig. 1.15)

(1)   external focusing
(2)   internal focusing
(3)   focusing mirror
(4)   electronic focusing = phased array
 → dynamic variable focusing
 → adjustable by sonographer
 → better resolution

Arrays

Array = collection of active elements in one TX
  (single slab of PZT-5 cut into small pieces)

Each active element is connected to its own electronic circuitry

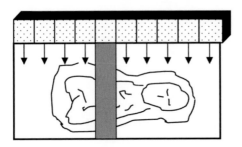

Fig. 1.16

Linear = elements in a line: linear switched array
linear phased array

Annular = elements with a common centre in a ring

Convex (curved) = collection in curved manner
  convex switched array
  convex linear array

Linear switched array (Fig. 1.16)
Large TX with elements arranged in a line
Image no wider than TX with a rectangular image
P/E crystals fire in sequence to give 2-D image
No steering/fixed vertical focusing
Defective crystal causes vertical dropout

Phased arrays (Fig. 1.17)
Collection of electric pulses delivered to the active elements in various
  patterns, which focus and steer U/S pulse
Fan-shaped image
Many signals excite multiple crystals → one sound pulse
If one element breaks → erratic focusing/steering
Small time delays (nearly simultaneous) between electronic pulses
  delivered to array elements

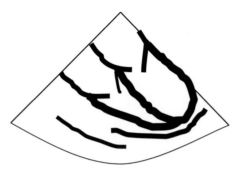

Fig. 1.17

Time delays during reception applied to electrical signals returning
   from TX to machine
'Reception zone' focusing can be matched to depth of returning echoes
   and optimizes image quality
Electronic curvature → focusing
Electronic slope → steering (Fig. 1.18)

Annular phased arrays
Concentric rings cut from circular slab of PZT-5
Small diameter → shallow focus (↓FD) and rapid divergence
Large diameter → ↑FD

Selected focal zones:
   inner crystals → shallow focus
   outer crystals → deep focus

Fan-shaped image
Electronic focusing/mechanical steering
Defective crystal causes horizontal dropout (Fig. 1.19)

Convex curved array (Fig. 1.20)
P/E crystals in curve → natural sector shape

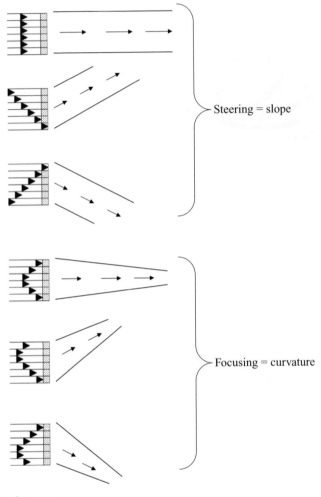

Fig. 1.18

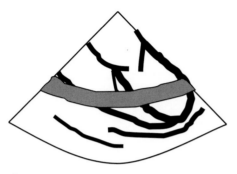

Fig. 1.19

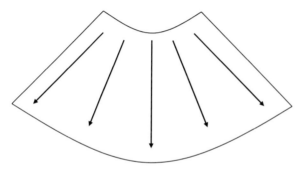

Fig. 1.20

Convex switched:
   sequential (large TX)
   no steering/fixed focusing
   defective crystal → vertical dropout

Blunted-fan image
Convex phased (small TX): electronic steering and focusing

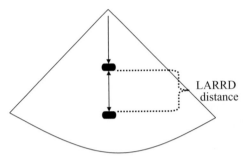

LARRD distance

Fig. 1.21

Imaging

Resolution

Longitudinal resolution

Longitudinal
Axial
Range   } **LARRD** resolution
Radial
Depth

Ability to distinguish two reflectors as separate entities parallel to U/S
   beam (Fig. 1.21)
Determined by source (f) and medium (λ)
TOE   LARRD = 0.05–0.5 mm

Improve LARRD resolution (i.e. ↓LARRD distance) by:
– ↑f→ ↓λ → ↓SPL → ↓LARRD distance
– ↓ringing → ↓SPL → ↓LARRD distance

$$\text{LARRD (mm)} = \text{SPL}/2$$

$$\text{LARRD (mm)} = 0.77 \times \text{ringing}/f \text{ (MHz)}$$

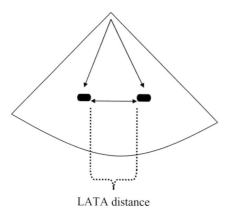

LATA distance

Fig. 1.22

Lateral resolution

Lateral
Angular   } **LATA**
Transverse   resolution
Azimuthal

Ability to distinguish two reflectors as separate entities perpendicular to
   U/S beam (Fig. 1.22)
LATA depends on beam width
LATA better when beam narrow
LATA optimal at FD (beam narrowest)
LATA varies with depth
When two reflectors are closer together than beam width, only one
   object is seen on image
LATA distance > LARRD distance (i.e. LARRD resolution is better than
   LATA resolution) because beam width > SPL
↑A/P/I → ↑LATA distance (i.e. degrades LATA resolution)

Temporal resolution
= frame rate, i.e. number of frames per second
1 pulse → 1 scan line → 1 image line

100 lines/frame = 100 pulses/frame → 1 picture
Not true for multiple focus beam systems and colour imaging because
    multiple pulses needed per scan line

Factors affecting temporal resolution

(1) number of pulses/scan line
(2) max. imaging depth
(3) sector size
(4) line density (lines/angle of sector)

↑ frame rate (better temporal resolution) by

(1) single focus, i.e. 1 pulse/scan line
(2) shallower image depth
(3) reduce sector size
(4) reduce line density

↓ frame rate (worse temporal resolution) by

(1) multifocus, e.g. colour flow imaging
(2) increase image depth, e.g. 6 cm → 12 cm → $\frac{1}{2}$ frame rate
(3) increase sector size
(4) increase line density

TOE temporal resolution = 30–60 frames/second on 2-D image
                          < 15 frames/second → 'flickering'

Display modes

A Mode (Fig. 1.23)
= amplitude mode
U/S pulse emitted → 'dot' moves across screen at constant speed
Echo returns → upward deflection of 'dot' proportional to amplitude
    of echo

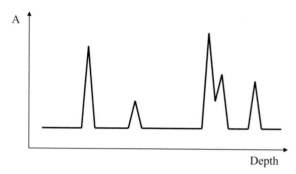

Fig. 1.23

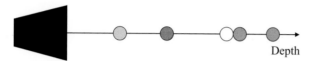

Fig. 1.24

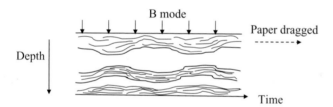

Fig. 1.25

B Mode (Fig. 1.24)

= brightness mode

Returning echoes appear as 'spots' on line of travel of emitted U/S pulse

Brightness of 'spot' proportional to amplitude

M Mode (Fig. 1.25)

= motion mode

Dragging photosensitive paper across B mode creates lines instead of dots, giving motion of reflected surfaces occurring in time

High temporal resolution $= 1000\times/$second

Ideal for imaging localized areas of heart and analysing time-related events

2-D imaging

Multiple narrow beams of pulsed U/S

B mode can be moved through path by sonographer to create 2-D picture, but slow and patient movement causes artefacts

Real-time imaging

U/S system steers beam through pathway

Multiple scan lines gives 2-D image at 30–60 frames/s

3-D echo

Requires:

    sequential acquisition of 2-D data from multiple planes

    digitization of data and off-line reconstruction

      Time-consuming

Instrumentation

Six components:

    Transducer (TX)

    Pulser

    Receiver

    Display

    Storage

    Master synchronizer (M/S)

Transducer

Transmission: electrical → acoustic energy

Reception: acoustic → electrical energy

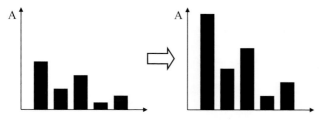

Fig. 1.26

Pulser

Controls electrical signals sent to TX for pulse generation

Receives signal from M/S

Determines:

   PRF/PRP

   Amplitude ($\uparrow$voltage $\to$ $\uparrow A$)

   Firing pattern for phased array TX

CW: constant electrical sine wave signal

PW (single crystal): one electrical 'spike' $\to$ one pulse

PW (arrays): many 'spikes' $\to$ one pulse

Receiver

Signals returning back from TX are weak

Therefore, needs 'boosting', 'processing' and 'preparing' for display

(1)   Amplification

   $\uparrow$Gain $\to$ every signal amplified (Fig. 1.26)

   Changed by sonographer

(2)   Compensation

   Attenuation proportional to image depth

   Deep image $\to$ $\downarrow A$

Changed by sonographer

(1) Time-gain compensation (TGC) = 'depth' compensation

   Amplifies signal from deeper objects (Fig. 1.27)

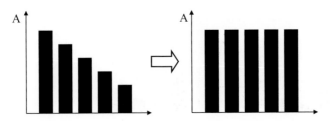

Fig. 1.27

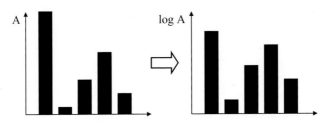

Fig. 1.28

(2) Lateral gain compensation (LGC) = 'lateral' compensation
    Allows application of gain to selected sectors
(3) Compression = dynamic range manipulation (Fig. 1.28)
    Process of reducing total range of received echo amplitudes
    Keeps signal within operating range
    Does not alter relationship between voltages
    Converts linear scale to log scale → uniformity of signals
(4) Demodulation
    Changes signal into form suitable for display
    'Rectification' = negative to positive voltage
    'Enveloping' = 'smoothing' of signal
    'Leading edge enhancement' = narrower and brighter image
(5) Rejection = filtering (Fig. 1.29)
    Low A signals associated with 'noise' rejected

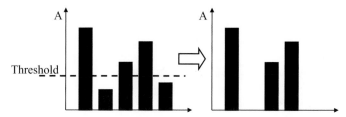

Fig. 1.29

Display

Cathode ray tubes (CRT) = TV screens (525 horizontal lines)

Electron beam strikes phosphor coating on screen → light

(1) interlaced: odd number lines filled in first, then even

(2) non-interlaced: lines filled in sequentially

Storage

Cine memory – captures short sequences in digital memory

Videotape – analog format

DVD – 1 frame = 1 Mbyte, large memory needed

Master synchronizer

Communicates with all components and organizes

Doppler

Principles

Doppler effect:

    The frequency of a sound wave reflected by a moving object is different
from that emitted

    = frequency shift/Doppler frequency (f_D)

The magnitude and direction of f_D is related to the velocity and
direction of the moving object (Fig. 1.30)

$$f_D = 2 \, v f_O \cos \theta / c$$

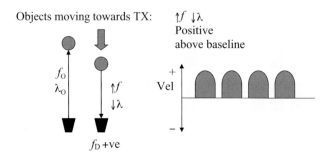

Objects moving towards TX: $\uparrow f \downarrow \lambda$
                               Positive
                               above baseline

f_D +ve

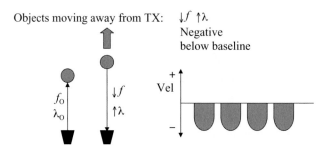

Objects moving away from TX: $\downarrow f \uparrow \lambda$
                                Negative
                                below baseline

Fig. 1.30

v = velocity of rbc
c = 1540 m/s
f_D = frequency shift
f_O = emitted frequency
θ = angle of incidence

Parallel beam ($0°$ and $180°$) $\rightarrow \cos \theta = 1$
Perpendicular beam ($90°$ and $270°$) $\rightarrow \cos \theta = 0$
Angle of incidence $< 20° \rightarrow < 6\%$ error
Measured velocity = true velocity $\times \cos \theta$

$$v = c \ f_D / 2 \ f_O \cos \theta$$

Unidirectional Doppler measures presence of moving rbc by Doppler shift, but cannot distinguish +ve or –ve, i.e. unidirectional

Bidirectional Doppler distinguishes +ve from −ve

TOE f_D = 20–20 000 Hz (i.e. audible)

Pulse wave Doppler

PW: one crystal emits and receives at specific PRF
    blood flow parameters at specific point (sample volume)

(1) mechanical sector scanners: TX stopped to record signal
(2) phased array:
        uses missing signal estimator (MSE)
        Doppler 'on' for 10 ms → Doppler signal
        2-D image 'on' for 20 ms→ 2-D image
        total time = 30 ms → 30 frames/second
        MSE gives synthesized signal during 2-D 20 ms
    Pulsed Doppler 'interrogates' target once per PRP
    Time delay (T_d), from emission of U/S beam to reception of signal,
        determines depth at which flow is sampled

   Depth = $c\,Td/2$

PWD = good for velocities < 2 m/s
Velocities > 2 m/s → 'aliasing' artefact

High pulse repetition frequency
= modification of PWD
2–5 samples simultaneously

Allows:
    ↑f because TX does not wait for return of signals before sending next
        pulse
    ↑max velocity before 'aliasing' occurs
    BUT – 'range ambiguity', i.e. do not know exactly where along pathway
        signal is returning from

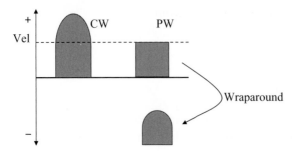

Fig. 1.31

'Aliasing'

When f_D exceeds certain limit, 'aliasing' (wraparound) occurs

High velocities appear negative (Fig. 1.31)

f_D at which aliasing occurs = Nyquist limit (frequency) = f_N

$$f_N = PRF/2$$

When $f_D > f_N \rightarrow$ 'aliasing'/wraparound artefact

Reduce aliasing by

    Use TX with $\downarrow f$

    Shallower depth (D) $\rightarrow$ $\uparrow$PRF

    Use CW

    Baseline shift

Max velocity (V_{max}) before aliasing occurs is given by:

$$V_{max}\ D = c^2/8\ f_O$$

$\downarrow f_O \rightarrow \uparrow V_{max} \rightarrow \downarrow$aliasing

$\downarrow$Depth $\rightarrow \uparrow V_{max}/\uparrow$PRF $\rightarrow \uparrow f_N \rightarrow \downarrow$aliasing

Continuous wave Doppler

CW uses two crystals:

    (1) transmitter

    (2) receiver

Allows high V_{max} (up to 9 m/s) without aliasing
BUT → 'range ambiguity'

PW	vs.	*CW*
(1) one crystal		two crystals
(2) range resolution		range ambiguity
(3) $V_{max} < 2$ m/s		V_{max} up to 9 m/s

Colour flow imaging

'Real-time' blood flow as colour on 2-D image
→ location, direction, velocity and laminar or turbulent flow

Based on multi-gated PWD, therefore:
   range resolution
   subject to aliasing

Multiple pulses → one Doppler packet → mean velocity of rbc
↑no. of pulses/packet → ↑accuracy of velocity
BUT ↑pulses/packet → ↓frame rate

Colour assigned to velocity depends on direction/flow type

Traditionally –
   red = towards TX
   blue = away from TX
   green hue (variance mode) = turbulence

LARRD vs. velocity resolution
Short SPL → better LARRD
Long SPL → better velocity resolution

Depth vs. PRF
Depth inversely proportional to PRF

Velocity resolution/depth/line density/frame rate

Many pulses down each line, averaged to give mean velocity

$$n \times \text{PRP} \times N \times F = 1$$

$n = $ pulses/line
$\text{PRP} = 1/\text{PRF}$
$N = $ lines/frame
$F = $ frame rate

Therefore, increase in one parameter leads to decrease in others

Tissue Doppler imaging (TDI)

Three modalities:
　Pulse wave-TDI (PW-TDI)
　2-dimensional-TDI (2-D-TDI)
　M mode-TDI (MM-TDI)

Sample volume placed on myocardium or A–V valve annulus
High frequency, low amplitude signals from blood filtered out
Measures peak velocities of a selected region
Mean velocities calculated to give colour velocity maps

PW-TDI

Good temporal resolution

Wave pattern:
　S wave (ventricular systole)
　IVRT
　E wave (rapid diastolic filling)
　Diastasis
　A wave (atrial contraction)

Tissue Doppler velocities $\approx$ 5–15 cm/s

2-D-TDI

Poor temporal resolution/good spatial resolution
Uses colour flow imaging
Low velocity myocardium coded with dark colours
High velocity myocardium coded with lighter colours

MM-TDI

Excellent temporal resolution
Uses colour flow imaging with M mode

Artefacts

Reverberations

Secondary reflection along the path of the U/S pulse due to the U/S
  'bouncing' between the structure and another strong reflector or the
  transducer
Creates parallel irregular lines at successively greater depths from the
  primary target
Two types (Fig. 1.32)
 (i) linear reverberation
 (ii) ring down = solid line directed away from TX due to merging of
  reverberations

Ghosting

Type of reverberation artefact when using colour flow Doppler
  (Fig. 1.33)
Amplitude of 'ghost' > A of initial reflector if target is moving

Mirror images

Occurs with Doppler (CW and PW)
↑↑ A of f_D spectrum → signal in opposite direction (normally below
  threshold, therefore filtered out) exceeds threshold (Fig. 1.34)

(a)

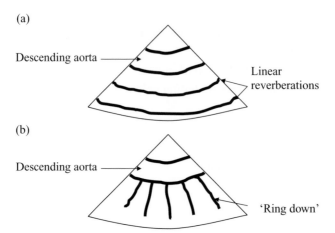

Descending aorta

Linear reverberations

(b)

Descending aorta

'Ring down'

Fig. 1.32

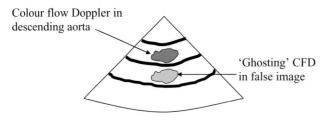

Colour flow Doppler in descending aorta

'Ghosting' CFD in false image

Fig. 1.33

Aliasing

= 'wraparound'

With PWD, when f_D exceeds Nyquist limit (Fig. 1.35)

$$f_D > PRF/2$$

Usually > 2 m/s

Reduced by:

   (1) $\downarrow f_O$

   (2) $\uparrow PRF$ ($\downarrow$depth)

   (3) use CWD

   (4) baseline shift

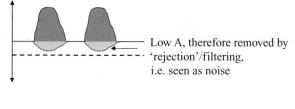

Low A, therefore removed by
'rejection'/filtering,
i.e. seen as noise

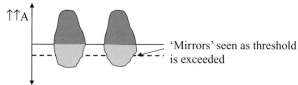

'Mirrors' seen as threshold
is exceeded

Fig. 1.34

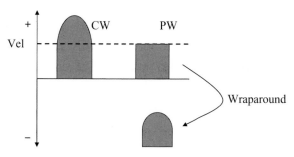

Wraparound

Fig. 1.35

Shadowing

U/S beam hits a strong reflector (e.g. mechanical valve)
→ ↓↓A of beam distal to reflector
→ 'fallout', i.e. no image seen beyond reflector

'Enhancement' = reverse shadowing
U/S beam hits very weak reflector with minimal attenuation
→ ↑reflection from distal tissue
→ brighter image (corrected using TGC)

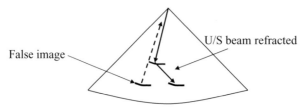

False image

U/S beam refracted

Fig. 1.36

Near field clutter

In the 'near field' strong signals are received from reflectors, which dominate the image

Amplitude of near field echoes reduced by: near field gain control

Refraction

U/S beam is deflected from its path
Creates falsely perceived object (Fig. 1.36)
TX assumes reflected signal originated from original scan line

Range ambiguity

With CWD: unsure of exact site of peak velocity/f_D along the U/S beam path
With high PRF: unsure from which of the several sites the signal may be returning.

Side lobes

TX emits several side beams with the main central beam
Reflection from side beam appears as object in main beam
Usually, multiple side lobes create a curved line, with the true reflector the brightest (Fig. 1.37)

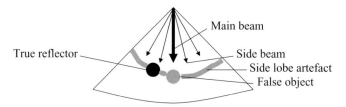

Fig. 1.37

Have common radius from TX
Cross anatomical planes

Beam width

= spatial resolution problem occurring with Doppler
↑ beam width → poor LATA
↑ beam width → inappropriate spatial localization
i.e. strong flow signals at margin of beam appear to arise from central
  part of beam

'Crying'

f_D in audible range (20–20 000 Hz)
TX acts as a microphone
External noise (e.g. patient talking) with high A is detected by TX,
causing oversaturation of amplifier
'Noise' displayed on spectral image

Multiple choice questions

1. The speed of sound through the heart is approximately
    A. 330 m/s
    B. 1450 m/s
    C. 1540 m/s

D. 14.5 mm/μs

E. 1.54 cm/μs

2. Audible sound has a frequency of

  A 2–20 Hz

  B 20–20 000 Hz

  C 20–20 000 kHz

  D 2–20 MHz

  E >20 MHz

3 The speed of sound through a medium is increased with

  A increased transducer frequency

  B increased medium density

  C reduced medium stiffness

  D increased medium bulk modulus

  E increased medium elasticity

4 The following are all acoustic variables except

  A density

  B force

  C temperature

  D pressure

  E particle motion

5 The intensity of an ultrasound wave is

  A measured in watts

  B the concentration of power in a beam

  C amplitude multiplied by power

  D amplitude squared

  E usually less than 100 mW

6 In pulsed ultrasound, pulse duration is

  A determined by the period of each cycle

  B analogous to wavelength

  C 0.5–3 seconds in TOE

  D number of cycles multiplied by frequency

  E altered by the sonographer

7 At a depth of 10 cm, the pulse repetition frequency is
   A 3.75 Hz
   B 7.5 Hz
   C 3.75 kHz
   D 7.5 kHz
   E 7500 kHz

8 When the pulse repetition period is 0.104 seconds, the depth of the image is
   A 4 cm
   B 5 cm
   C 6 cm
   D 7 cm
   E 8 cm

9 Spatial pulse length
   A influences axial resolution
   B influences lateral resolution
   C is usually 0.1–1 μm in TOE
   D is determined only by the medium
   E is changed by the sonographer

10 The following are true regarding attenuation except
   A it occurs by absorption
   B it can be measured in decibels
   C it increases with reducing transducer frequency
   D it occurs by scattering
   E it occurs by reflections

11 With a 6 MHz ultrasound transducer, the half value layer thickness is
   A 1 mm
   B 0.5 cm
   C 1 cm
   D 1.5 cm
   E 3 cm

12 All the following statements are true except
   A in soft tissue acoustic impedance is 1.25–1.75 Rayls
   B reflections depend upon changes in acoustic impedance

    C acoustic impedance is density multiplied by velocity

    D specular reflections occur at smooth boundaries

    E acoustic impedance is resistance to sound propagation

13 The intensity reflection coefficient of a sound wave traveling from medium 1 ($Z = 20$ Rayls) to medium 2 ($Z = 80$ Rayls) is

    A 30–40%

    B 40–50%

    C 50–60%

    D 60–70%

    E 70–80%

14 With regard to ultrasound transducers

    A TOE transducers have a frequency of 3–6 Hz

    B each piezoelectric crystal is supplied by four electrical wires

    C most ultrasound crystals are made from quartz

    D the damping element improves temporal resolution

    E the matching layer has a lower impedance than the crystal

15 The following statements about sound beams are true except

    A the focus is the position of minimum diameter

    B the Fresnel zone is the near zone

    C smaller diameter transducers have a shorter focal depth

    D higher frequency transducers have a shorter focal depth

    E smaller diameter transducers have greater divergence

16 Axial resolution is

    A improved by reduced ringing

    B worsened by increasing transducer frequency

    C improved by increasing spatial pulse length

    D worsened by shortening wavelength

    E the ability to separate two objects perpendicular to the beam

17 Temporal resolution can be improved by

    A increasing image depth

    B adding colour flow Doppler to the image

    C adding pulse wave Doppler to the image

    D reducing sector size

    E increasing line density

18 Motion (M) mode imaging
  A requires sequential acquisition from multiple planes
  B has low temporal resolution
  C has velocity on the y-axis
  D is poor for analysing time-related events
  E is developed from B mode imaging

19 Pulse wave Doppler
  A suffers from 'range ambiguity' artefact
  B requires one crystal to emit and a second crystal to receive
  C is used in colour flow Doppler imaging
  D is accurate with velocities up to 9 m/s
  E suffers from 'aliasing' at velocities above 2 cm/s

20 The following statements regarding 'aliasing' are true except
  A it is reduced by imaging at a shallower depth
  B it is worsened by increasing transducer frequency
  C it can be removed by changing to pulse wave Doppler
  D it is reduced by increasing pulse repetition frequency
  E it occurs when the Doppler frequency exceeds the Nyquist limit

2

Guidelines and safety

Indications

Category I

TOE useful in improving clinical outcomes

(1) Pre-operative
   (a) suspected TAA, dissection or disruption in unstable patient
(2) Intra-operative
   (a) life-threatening haemodynamic disturbance
   (b) valve repair
   (c) congenital heart surgery
   (d) HOCM repair
   (e) endocarditis
   (f) AV function in aortic dissection repair
   (g) evaluation of pericardial window procedures
(3) ICU setting
   (a) unexplained haemodynamic disturbances

Category II

TOE may be useful in improving clinical outcomes

(1) Pre-operative
   (a) suspected TAA, dissection or disruption in stable patient
(2) Intra-operative
   (a) valve replacement

(b) cardiac aneurysm repair

(c) cardiac tumour excision

(d) detection of foreign bodies

(e) detection of air emboli during cardiac/neuro procedures

(f) intracardiac thrombectomy

(g) pulmonary embolectomy

(h) suspected cardiac trauma

(i) aortic dissection repair

(j) aortic atheromatous disease/source of aortic emboli

(k) pericardial surgery

(l) anastomotic sites during heart/lung transplant

(m) placement of assist devices

(3) Peri-operative

(a) increased risk of haemodynamic disturbances

(b) increased risk of myocardial ischaemia

Category III

TOE infrequently useful in improving clinical outcomes

(1) Intra-operative

(a) evaluation of myocardial perfusion, coronary artery anatomy, or graft patency

(b) repair of non-HOCM cardiomyopathies

(c) endocarditis in non-cardiac surgery

(d) monitoring emboli in orthopaedic surgery

(e) repair of thoracic aortic injuries

(f) uncomplicated pericarditis

(g) pleuropulmonary disease

(h) monitoring cardioplegia administration

(2) Peri-operative

(a) placement of IABP, ICD or PA catheters

Safety

Contraindications and complications

Absolute contraindications

(1) patient refusal

(2) patient has had oesophagectomy

(3) recent major oesophageal surgery

(4) oesophageal atresia, stricture, tumour

Relative contraindications

(1) oesophageal diverticulum

(2) oesophageal varices

(3) Barrett's oesophagus

(4) recent oesophageal/gastric radiotherapy

(5) hiatus hernia

(6) unexplained upper gastrointestinal bleed

(7) in awake patient where tachycardia undesirable

Complications

Minor < 13%   Serious < 3%

Mortality 0.01–0.03%

(1) direct trauma to:
     mouth: lip, dental injuries
     pharynx: sore throat
     larynx: RLN injury, tracheal insertion (!)
     oesophagus: dysphagia, tear, burn
     stomach: haemorrhage

(2) indirect effects:
     tachycardia, causing myocardial ischaemia
     bradycardia
     arrhythmias
     bacteraemia

(3) equipment damage

Biological effects

Dosimetry $=$ science of identifying/measuring characteristics of ultrasound fields causing biological effects

High A/P/I causes damage (SPTA related to tissue heating)
SPTA < 100 mW/cm^2 unfocused $=$ safe
SPPA < 1 W/cm^2 focused $=$ safe

Thermal

Tissue absorption (bone) of U/S $\rightarrow$ heat
Localized scattering $\rightarrow$ heat
TOE exam causing $< 1\,°C$ rise in temperature $=$ safe
$\qquad\qquad\qquad\quad > 41\,°C \rightarrow$ harmful
Tightly focused beams $\rightarrow \uparrow$ temperature elevation as heat is dissipated
Unfocused beams $\rightarrow \downarrow$ temperature elevation
Fetal $\uparrow$ temperature a concern (effects on fetal bone)
Thermal index $=$ quantification of tissue heating

Cavitation

Bodies of gas/microbubbles are excited by U/S
$\rightarrow$ vibration $\rightarrow$ tissue and heat injury

(1) stable cavitation

$\quad$ oscillating bubbles: $\left.\begin{array}{l} \text{intercept} \\ \text{reradiate} \\ \text{absorb} \end{array}\right\}$ acoustic energy

$\quad \rightarrow$ shear stresses/microstreaming in surrounding fluid

(2) transient cavitation

$\quad$ bubbles expand and burst $\rightarrow$ highly localized violent effects
$\quad$ mechanical index $=$ quantification of cavitation effects

Electrical hazards

Uncommon

Patient susceptible to electrical injury from:

(1) frayed/worn cables
(2) damaged U/S TX
(3) damaged case/housing
(4) damaged electrical circuitry/plug

Infection

Incidence of bacteraemia is up to 4%

but no evidence for clinical consequences
Antibiotic prophylaxis only recommended in high risk patients

Infectious complications reduced by:

(1) use of mouth guard
(2) careful insertion/removal of probe
(3) gross decontamination
(4) Hibiscrub wash
(5) soak in Metiricide > 20 min
(6) rinse in water

Multiple choice questions

1. The following are category I indications for TOE except
   A mitral valve repair
   B congenital heart surgery
   C life-threatening haemodynamic disturbances
   D evaluation of pericardial window procedures
   E cardiac tumour excision
2. An absolute contraindication to perioperative TOE is
   A oesophageal atresia
   B Barrett's oesophagus
   C hiatus hernia

    D unexplained upper gastrointestinal bleed

    E oesophageal diverticulum

3. The following statements relating to the biological effects of ultrasound are true except

    A tightly focused beams cause less of a temperature rise

    B TOE is considered safe if temperature rises less then 1 °C

    C in transient cavitation, bubbles expand and burst

    D thermal index is the quantification of tissue heating

    E focused beams are considered safe if the intensity is less than 1 kW/cm^2

4. With regard to complications of TOE

    A bacteraemia occurs in 15% of patients

    B serious complications occur in 5–10% of patients

    C indirect complications include tachyarrhythmias

    D mortality from TOE is 0.1%

    E antibiotic prophylaxis is recommended for all patients

3

Normal anatomy and physiology

Chambers

Left atrium (Fig. 3.1)

LA area $= 14.0 \text{ cm}^2 \pm 3 \text{ cm}^2$
LA pressure $= 2\text{--}10 \text{ mmHg}$
LA $SaO_2 = 97\%$

LA appendage

Seen at $30°\text{--}150°$
Single or multiple lobes
May contain pectinate muscles
Common site for thrombus

Doppler velocities:
    contraction (emptying) and filling
    low velocities associated with thrombus

Right atrium (Fig. 3.2)

RA area $= 13.5 \text{ cm}^2 \pm 2 \text{ cm}^2$
RA pressure $= 1\text{--}5 \text{ mmHg}$
RA $SaO_2 = 75\%$

Left ventricle (Fig. 3.3)

LV pressure $= 120/10$
LV $SaO_2 = 97\%$
LV FS% (Mmode) $\approx 30\text{--}45\%$

Four-chamber view

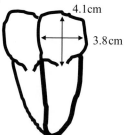

4.1 cm

3.8 cm

Fig. 3.1

Four-chamber view

4.2 cm

3.7 cm

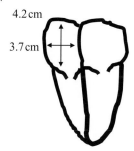

Fig. 3.2

(a) Four-chamber view

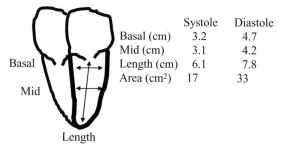

Basal

Mid

Length

	Systole	Diastole
Basal (cm)	3.2	4.7
Mid (cm)	3.1	4.2
Length (cm)	6.1	7.8
Area (cm^2)	17	33

(b) Short axis view

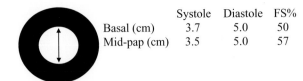

	Systole	Diastole	FS%
Basal (cm)	3.7	5.0	50
Mid-pap (cm)	3.5	5.0	57

Fig. 3.3a, b (*cont.*)

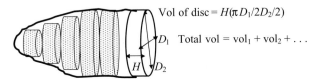

Vol of disc $= H(\pi D_1/2 D_2/2)$

Total vol $=$ vol$_1$ + vol$_2$ + . . .

Fig. 3.4

LV volume

LVEDV index $= 50$–$60 \, \mathrm{ml/m^2}$

Calculated using Simpson's method $=$ sum of volume of discs (Fig. 3.4)

LV segments

Midoesophageal views (Fig. 3.5)

Transgastric short axis views (Fig. 3.6)

Right ventricle (Fig. 3.7)

RV pressure $= 25/5 \, \mathrm{mmHg}$

RV SaO$_2$ $= 75\%$

RV FS% $= 45$–50%

RV volume

Determined by Simpson's method

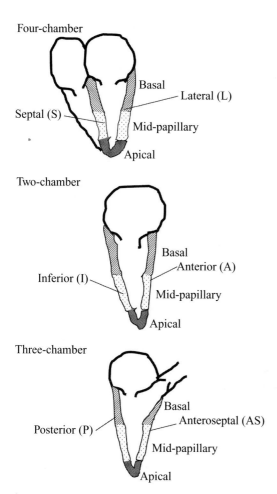

Four-chamber

Basal
Lateral (L)
Septal (S)
Mid-papillary
Apical

Two-chamber

Basal
Anterior (A)
Inferior (I)
Mid-papillary
Apical

Three-chamber

Basal
Anteroseptal (AS)
Posterior (P)
Mid-papillary
Apical

Fig. 3.5

Valves

Mitral valve

Two leaflets:
   anterior (AMVL)
   posterior (PMVL)

SAX basal

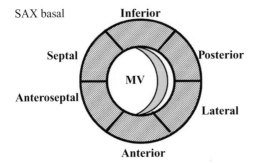

SAX mid-papillary

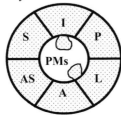

SAX apical

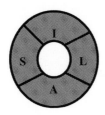

Fig. 3.6

Attachment of PMVL > AMVL
Size of AMVL > PMVL (Fig. 3.8)
Normal MV area (MVA) = 4–6 cm^2

Composed of:
    leaflets
    chordae tendineae
    papillary muscles (PMs)
    fibromuscular annulus

Four-chamber

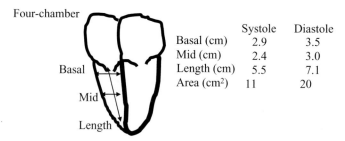

	Systole	Diastole
Basal (cm)	2.9	3.5
Mid (cm)	2.4	3.0
Length (cm)	5.5	7.1
Area (cm²)	11	20

Fig. 3.7

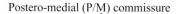
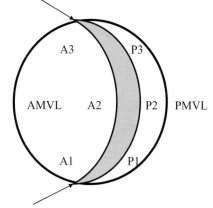

Fig. 3.8

From each PM – 1°/2°/3° chordal structures
　　　　　　subdivide and attach to ventricular surface and free
　　　　　　edge of AMVL and PMVL
Fibromuscular annulus supports PMVL
AMVL continuous with membranous ventricular septum, aortic valve,
　　and aorta
AMVL attaches to fibrous skeleton of heart
All aspects of AMVL and PMVL seen on midoesophageal views (Fig. 3.9)

(a) Four-chamber (0°)

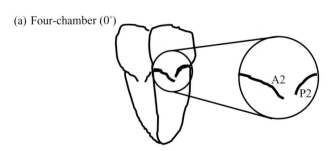

(b) Commissural (40–60°)

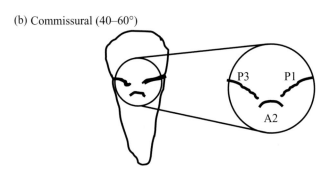

(c) Two-chamber (90°)

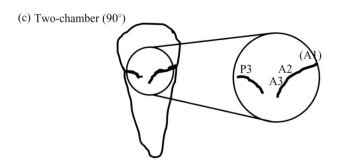

(d) Three-chamber (110–140°)

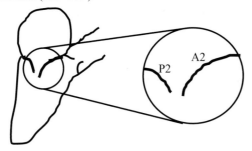

(e) Five-chamber (0° and anteflex)

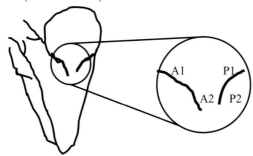

Fig. 3.9a, b, c, d, e (*cont.*)

MVL motion (Mmode) (Fig. 3.10)

D → E = early diastole/passive rapid LV filling

E → F = ↓LA pressure prior to LA contraction

F → A = atrial systole

A → C = LV pressure (LVP) > LA pressure (LAP) → trivial MR
          LV systole → LVP >> LAP → MV closes (MVC)

Factors affecting MVL motion

(1) LAP: LVP

(2) volume/velocity of blood flow across MV

(3) annulus/PM motion

(4) LA/LV compliance (Cn)

(5) LV systolic function

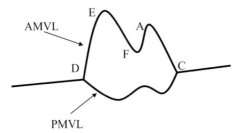

Fig. 3.10

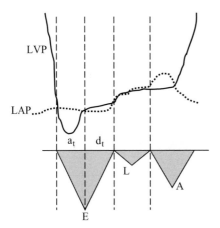

Fig. 3.11

Transmitral flow (TMF)

PW Doppler at MVL tips (Fig. 3.11)

E = passive LV filling: a_t due to LAP > LVP

d_t due to inertia of flow

L = pulmonary veins (PVs) filling LA → LAP > LVP

L incorporated into E as HR increases

A = atrial systole

Doppler velocities

E = 50–80 cm/s (decreases with increasing age)

A = 30–50 cm/s (increases with age/diastolic dysfunction)

E/A = 1–2.2/1 (ratio decreases with age)

VTI_E/VTI_A = 2.5/1

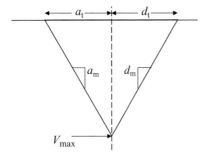

Fig. 3.12

E wave (Fig. 3.12)

a_m = flow acceleration

determined by rate of ↑pressure gradient (PG) when MVO

secondary to: initial LAP

rate of LV relaxation

MV resistance (MV area)

d_m = determined by rate of equalization of LAP:LVP

related to LA/LV Cn

i.e. ↓LV Cn → ↑rate of d_m (↓d_t)

d_t (deceleration time DT) = due to flow inertia

reduced MVA (e.g. MS) → ↑d_t

V_{max} determined by: initial LAP:LVP

LA/LV Cn

↑V_{max} with ↑LAP

↓V_{max} with ↓LV Cn

Aortic valve

Three leaflets:

left coronary cusp (LCC)

right coronary cusp (RCC)

non-coronary cusp (NCC)

with associated sinuses of Valsalva (Fig. 3.13)

(a) AV SAX (30–60°)

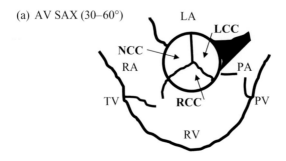

(b) AV LAX (110–140°)

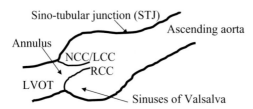

Fig. 3.13a, b

Leaflet = crescent-shaped

        thickening at leaflet tip = node of Arantius (↑ with age)

        two ridges from node to lateral margins = coaptation line

        above ridges = lunula (fenestrated)

Lambl's excrescences = filamentous lesions on free edge of leaflet

                connective tissue

                degenerative change

                ? nidus for infection/thrombus

Doppler flow (Fig. 3.14)

Normal flow = systolic

        laminar (some turbulence at peak systole)

        rapid acceleration

        peak at mid-systole

        slow deceleration

        AV closes

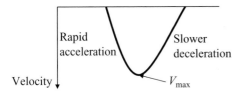

Fig. 3.14

TG SAX

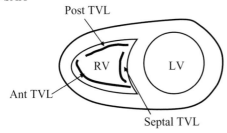

Fig. 3.15

Flow velocity depends on:
   CO
   SVR
   AV area

AV V_{max} = 1.35 m/s (1.0–1.7 m/s)
LVOT V_{max} = 0.9 m/s (0.7–1.1 m/s)

Tricuspid valve

Three leaflets: anterior (largest)
             posterior
             septal (Fig. 3.15)
PMs: anterior (largest) from moderator band
     posterior and septal (small)
TVL = continuous veil of fibrous tissue
        indentations = commissures

Septal TVL insertion infero-apical compared to anterior TVL

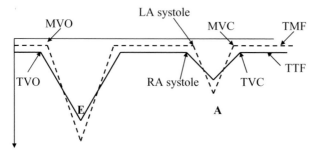

Fig. 3.16

Transtricuspid flow (TTF)

TV opens before MV because:

    peak RVP < LVP

    RAP > RVP before LAP > LVP

TV closes after MV because:

    LV activation before RV

    LVP > LAP before RVP > RAP

RA systole before LA systole (activated from SA node in RA)

TTF vs. TMF (Fig. 3.16)

a_m determined by:

    initial RAP

    rate of RV relaxation

    TV resistance (TVA)

d_m determined by:

    RA/RV Cn

    ↓ RV Cn → ↑ rate of d_m

TTF E V_{max} < TMF because RAP < LAP

TTF E a_m < TMF because RAP < LAP

TTF E d_m < TMF because RV Cn > LV Cn

Respiration

Greater influence on TTF compared to TMF

On inspiration → TTF increases

$\uparrow$E V_{max} and A V_{max} by $\approx$ 15%

E/A ratio remains constant

Pulmonary valve

Three leaflets: anterior

right posterior

left posterior

Lies anterior/superior/to the left of AV

PV area > AV area

Flow

Systolic

Laminar

Mid-systolic peak V_{max}

PV V_{max} = 0.6–0.9 m/s

Vessels

Aorta

Thick musculoelastic wall – thin intima

thick media, multiple elastic sheets

thin adventitia

Ascending aorta (Fig. 3.17)

From AV to aortic arch $\approx$ 5 cm

Commences at AV at LSE third CC

Passes anterior/superior/to the right

Joins proximal aortic arch at RSE second CC

Branches:

LCA from LC sinus

RCA from RC sinus

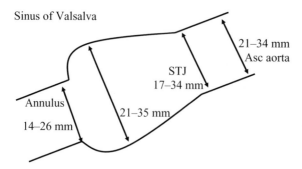

Fig. 3.17

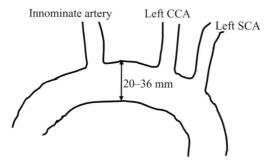

Fig. 3.18

Aortic arch (Fig. 3.18)

Runs from ascending aorta to descending aorta

Commences at RSE second CC

Initially passes superior/posterior/lateral in front of trachea

Passes inferior/to the left

Joins descending aorta at anterior aspect of T4

Branches:

  innominate artery

  left common carotid artery

  left subclavian artery

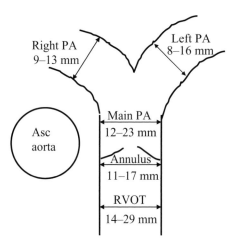

Fig. 3.19

Descending aorta

Commences at distal aortic arch

Runs from arch to iliac bifurcation at L4

Divided into thoracic and abdominal by diaphragm at T12

Thoracic aorta diameter ≈ 20 mm

Pulmonary artery

Runs from PV to bifurcation into LPA and RPA

Approximately 2–3 cm in length (Fig. 3.19)

LPA passes posteriorly/to the left, to left hilum

RPA passes to the right beneath aorta, superior branch passes to right hilum

Doppler flow

Laminar flow with flat velocity profile

Normal PA $= 0.6–0.9$ m/s

PA flow: ↑15% on inspiration

↑30% post-Fontan's procedure

↑50% with tamponade

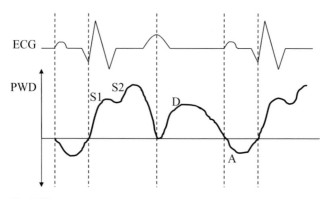

Fig. 3.20

Pulmonary veins

Four veins: 2 right–upper and lower (RUPV and RLPV)

2 left–upper and lower (LUPV and LLPV)

2% population have > 2 PVs from right lung

Doppler flow composed of S, D and A waves (Fig. 3.20)

S wave (PV$_S$)

Systolic antegrade flow due to low LAP

S1 = atrial relaxation

S2 = mitral annular plane systolic exclusion (MAPSE), due to the descent of MV annulus with LV systole

Affected by:

LA C_n

MR

Normal PV$_S$ = 40 cm/s

D wave (PV$_D$)

Diastolic antegrade flow due to drop in LAP when MV opens

Determined by PG from PV:LA

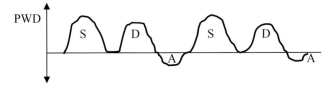

Fig. 3.21

Peak PV_D occurs 50 msec after peak E V_{max}
Normal $PV_D = 30$ cm/s

A wave (PV_A)

Diastolic retrograde flow due to atrial contraction
Reversal of flow back into PV depends on LV C_n
i.e. $\downarrow LV\ C_n \rightarrow \uparrow PV_A$ reversal
Normal $PV_A = 20$ cm/s
Atrial fibrillation (AF):
  no PV_{S1}
  no PV_A
  $PV_{S2} < PV_D$

Coronary sinus

Venous return of heart
Posterior aspect of heart in A–V groove
Covered by LA wall and pericardium
Normal CS < 10 mm diam

Doppler flow composed of S, D and A waves (Fig. 3.21)

CS dilated with:
  RV dysfunction
  increased RAP
  increased volume flow, e.g. persistent left SVC

(a)

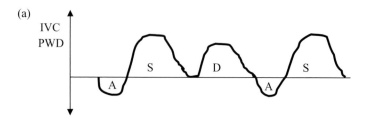

(b)

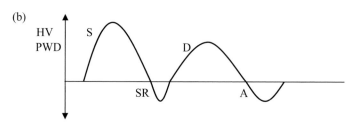

Fig. 3.22a, b

Vena cavae/hepatic veins

IVC

From common iliac veins at L5 to RA

Passes through diaphragm at T8/11–25 mm diameter

Doppler flow composed of S, D and A waves (Fig. 3.22(a))

SVC

From R and L innominate veins to RA at third CC

HVs

Insert into IVC proximal to diaphragm (at ~ 30°)/5–11mm diam

Doppler flow composed of S, SR, D and A waves (Fig. 3.22(b))

S wave: ↓RAP due to: atrial relaxation

                                TAPSE

SR wave: slight reversal of flow at end of RV systole

D wave: ↓RAP as TV opens

A wave: RA contraction → small reversal of flow

Coronary arteries

From sinuses of Valsalva

LCA = 10 mm long/3–10 mm diam
         bifurcates into LAD and LCx
    LAD supplies ant LV/ant $\frac{2}{3}$ IVS

PWD of LAD during diastole = 40–70 cm/s

LCx supplies lat LV/SAN (40%)/AVN (15%)/post $\frac{1}{3}$ IVS

RCA supplies RA/RV/SAN (60%)/AVN (85%)/post $\frac{1}{3}$ IVS

Post $\frac{1}{3}$ IVS from post. desc. artery = RCA (50%)
                                        LCx (20%)
                                        RCA + LCx (30%)

Septa

Interatrial septum

Thin muscular membrane separating RA and LA

Depression in mid portion = fossa ovalis (foramen ovale in fetus)

Development (Fig. 3.23)

Downward growth of septum primum

Septum primum separates from superior atrium and continues
    downward growth

Downward growth of septum secundum to right of septum primum
    creates flap = foramen ovale (FO)

Fetus: RAP > LAP: FO open

Birth: LAP > RAP: FO closes

25% of population have patent FO (PFO)

IAS motion

Reflects RAP vs. LAP

Predominantly reflects LAP because LA less compliant than RA,
    therefore increase in volume increases LAP > RAP

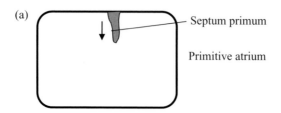

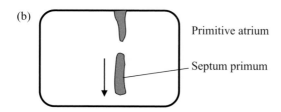

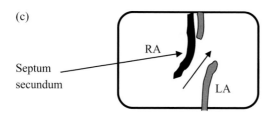

Fig. 3.23a, b, c

(1) movement to LA = RA contraction before LA systole
(2) movement to RA = LA filling
(3) continued movement to RA = TV opens before MV opens
(4) movement back to LA = MV opens, rapid LV filling

Interventricular septum

Thick, triangular muscular wall except small membranous part at
    superior border below AV (RCC and NCC)
Functional component of LV (= $\frac{1}{3}$ of LV muscle)

Concave to LV

Normal IVS = 7–12 mm thick (= LV free wall thickness)
(measured in mid-diastole)

Thin septum = post-MI scar tissue

<7 mm

high echogenicity

30% thinner than surrounding myocardium

IVS motion

Contracts with LV inwards towards centre of LV (SAX view)

Multiple choice questions

1. The normal left atrial area is
   A 4 mm^2
   B 1.4 cm^2
   C 4 cm^2
   D 10 cm^2
   E 14 cm^2
2. Normal right atrial oxygen saturation is
   A 55%
   B 65%
   C 75%
   D 85%
   E 95%
3. From the transgastric short axis view of the left ventricle, normal fractional shortening at basal level is
   A 20%
   B 35%
   C 50%
   D 65%
   E 80%

4. The left ventricular walls seen from the standard two chamber view (at 90°) are

A inferior and lateral

B anterior and lateral

C posterior and anteroseptal

D inferior and anterior

E septal and lateral

5. Normal right ventricular systolic and diastolic pressures are approximately

A 20/10 mmHg

B 25/5 mmHg

C 35/15 mmHg

D 25/15 mmHg

E 40/0 mmHg

6. The following statements about the normal mitral valve are all true except

A the posterior leaflet is continuous with the membranous ventricular septum

B the anterior leaflet is larger than the posterior leaflet

C there is an anterolateral and a posteromedial commissure

D chordal structures arise from the papillary muscles and attach to the ventricular surface of both the anterior and posterior leaflets

E the anterior leaflet attaches to the fibrous skeleton of the heart

7. The following parts of the mitral valve can be observed from the standard commissural view (at 40–60°)

A A1, A2, P1

B A2, P1, P3

C A1, A3, P2

D A1, P1, P2

E A3, P1, P3

8. Normal mitral valve area is

A 1–2 cm²

B 2–4 cm²

C 4–6 cm²

D 6–8 cm^2

E 10–14 cm^2

9. Regarding transmitral flow, a normal E wave velocity in a healthy 50-year-old is

A 3 cm/s

B 6 cm/s

C 30 cm/s

D 60 cm/s

E 3 m/s

10. The following statements regarding transmitral flow are all true except

A the E wave represents passive left ventricular filling

B the L wave occurs in late passive diastole

C the E wave duration is affected by left ventricular compliance

D the A wave velocity increases with increasing age

E the E wave velocity increases with increasing age

11. The normal aortic valve comprises the following three coronary cusps

A left, right and anterior

B left, right and posterior

C anterior, posterior and non-

D superior, inferior and non-

E left, right and non-

12. The normal maximum velocity measured by Doppler through the left ventricular outflow tract is

A 9 cm/s

B 90 cm/s

C 1.35 m/s

D 9 m/s

E 13.5 m/s

13. The following statements regarding the normal tricuspid valve are all true except

A it is composed of anterior, posterior, and septal leaflets

B the anterior leaflet insertion is infero-apical compared to the septal leaflet insertion

    C the tricuspid valve opens before the mitral valve opens

    D the tricuspid valve closes after the mitral valve closes

    E transtricuspid blood flow increases on inspiration

14. The normal diameter of the ascending aorta at the sino-tubular junction is

    A 14–26 mm

    B 17–34 mm

    C 21–35 mm

    D 25–41 mm

    E 26–41 mm

15. Regarding pulmonary venous Doppler flow waves

    A S2 is due to mitral annular plane systolic excursion

    B normal S wave velocity is 4 cm/s

    C D wave is due to atrial systole

    D normal D wave velocity is 30 m/s

    E A wave velocity decreases with reduced left ventricular compliance

16. Normal interventricular septum thickness measured in mid-diastole is

    A 1–2 mm

    B 2–5 mm

    C 5–7 mm

    D 7–12 mm

    E 12–17 mm

4

Ventricular function

LV systolic function

Quantitative echo

LV volume
Normal LVEDV $= 50$–$60 \, \text{ml}/\text{m}^2$
Calculated using Simpson's method (Fig. 3.4)

LV mass
LV adapts to increases in pressure and volume with muscular
   hypertrophy
Eccentric hypertrophy due to $\uparrow$ chamber volume (volume overload)
Concentric hypertrophy due to $\uparrow$ wall thickness
   (pressure overload)

$$\text{LV mass (LVM)} \approx V_{\text{ep}} - V_{\text{end}} = V_{\text{m}}$$

(i.e. LVM $=$ total within epicardium – total within endocardium)

LVM $= V_{\text{m}} \times 1.05$ (specific gravity for myocardium)
LVH is $> 134 \, \text{g}/\text{m}^2$ for men
   $> 120 \, \text{g}/\text{m}^2$ for women

Ejection indices
(1) Stroke volume   SV $=$ LVEDN $-$ LVESV
      SV index (SVI) $= 40$–$50 \, \text{ml}/\text{m}^2$

(2) Ejection fraction $EF = [(LVEDV - LVESV) / LVEDV] \times 100$

$EF = (SV/LVEDV) \times 100$

$EF = 50\text{–}70\%$

(3) Fractional shortening

$FS = [(LVIDd - LVIDs) / LVIDd] \times 100$

LVIDd = LV internal diameter in diastole

LVIDs = LV internal diameter in systole

$FS = 28\text{–}45\%$

(4) Velocity of circumferential fibre shortening (Vcf)

$Vcf = (LVIDd - LVIDs) / (LVIDd \times ET)$

ET = ejection time

Reflects amplitude and rate of LV contraction

$V_{cf} > 1.1$ circumferences/s

Global LV function

Contractility = thickening and inward movement of LV wall during systole

Quantitative assessment:

LV volume

>LV mass

>EF

>FS

>Vcf

Qualitative assessment:

>normal

>hypokinesia

>akinesia

>dyskinesia

Non-TOE assessment

(1) MRI: high resolution, 3-D images

    LV function, extent of ischaemia

(2) Nuclear imaging: myocardial scintigraphy (Tec-99)

    = 'hot-spot' imaging

    perfusion scintigraphy (Th-201)

    = 'cold-spot' imaging

    radionuclide angiography (Tec-99)

    = assesses LV function, CO, EF, and LVEDV

(3) CT scan: with Th-201

    perfusion defects, MI size

(4) Angiography: LV function

    coronary artery assessment

Effect of altered physiology/pathophysiology

(1) Exercise

    ↑HR ↑SV → ↑CO ↑EF ↑BP

    with LVESV↓/LVEDV↔

(2) AI

    ↑LVEDV/↑LVESV → ↑LVM (eccentric hypertrophy)

    EF remains normal until late (due to ↓SVR)

    Poor prognosis if LVIDs > 50 mm

(3) AS

    ↑LVM (concentric hypertrophy)

    ↑EF/↑V_{cf}

    ↓EF late in disease

(4) MR

    ↑LVEDV/↑LVESV → ↑LVM (eccentric hypertrophy)

    EF preserved until late in disease

    Poor prognosis if: LVIDs > 50 mm

      LVIDd > 70 mm

      FS < 30%

(5) Hypertension

    ↑wall stress

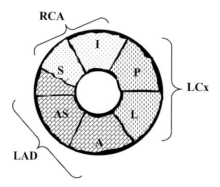

Fig. 4.1

↑LVM (concentric hypertrophy)
Diastolic dysfunction with ↑IVRT
(6) HOCM
Diagnosis: septum/post wall thickness > 1.3/1
This occurs in:
12% of normal population
32% of LV hypertrophy
95% of HOCM

Segmental LV function

Regional wall motion abnormality (RWMA)
Occurs 5–10 beats after coronary artery occlusion
Precedes ECG changes

Adjacent area asynergy = hypokinesia due to:

(1) mechanical tethering by ischaemic tissue
(2) ATP depletion
(3) metabolic abnormalities

Region of hypokinesia depends on blood supply (Fig. 4.1)
Other causes of RWMA:

(1) LBBB
(2) RBBB
(3) pacing
(4) WPW syndrome
(5) post-CPB

Chronic ischaemia

(1) Fixed RWMA: varies in size/distribution
(2) Scar: post-MI = dense and thin (<7 mm)
(3) Aneurysm: post-MI, traumatic, congenital
   (a) True: gradual expansion
      thinning of myocardium
      wide neck (> $^1/_2$ diam of aneurysm)
      assoc. with thrombus, arrhythmias, CCF
   (b) Pseudo:
      due to myocardial rupture
      blood contained by parietal pericardium
      narrow neck (< $^1/_2$ diam of aneurysm)
      assoc. with thrombus, rupture, arrhythmias, CCF
(4) VSD: post-MI IVS rupture with poor prognosis
(5) PM rupture: P/M PM more common than A/L PM causes
     severe MR
(6) Thrombus:
     common after large MI
     assoc. with LV aneurysm
     echo dense speckled mass
     interrupts LV contour
     common in apical aneurysms

Stress echo

Designed to induce RWMA by:
   exercise (treadmill)
   pharmacology (Dobutamine)
   pacing (transoesophageal)

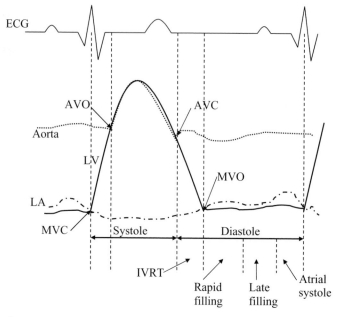

Fig. 4.2

Normal response = hyperkinesis/↑EF%/↑aortic VTI
Abnormal = new RWMA/worsening of existing RWMA/↓EF%

LV diastolic function

Phases of diastole (Fig. 4.2)

Isovolumic relaxation time (IVRT)
= 70–90 ms
From AVC – MVO
Aortic pressure > LVP → AV closes
LVP > LAP so MV remains closed
LV volume constant
LV relaxes → ↓LVP
IVRT ends when LAP > LVP & MV opens

Early rapid filling
= E wave on TMF
LAP >> LVP with continued LV relaxation
As LV fills → ↑LV vol → ↑LVP
As LAP LVP → ↓filling rate
As LAP = LVP → filling stops

Diastasis/late filling
= L wave on TMF
LAP LVP → little filling
PVs contribute to LV filling

Atrial systole
= A wave on TMF
↑LAP → LV filling (10–30% of total)

Indices of relaxation

IVRT
AVC – MVO
↓relaxation → ↑IVRT > 90 ms
    Affected by: aortic diastolic pressure (aortic DBP)
              LAP
i.e. ↓Aortic DBP/↑LAP → ↓IVRT

−dP/dt
Negative rate of change of LVP (Fig. 4.3)
Occurs soon after AVC
Affected by aortic systolic pressure (aortic SBP)
i.e. ↑Aortic SBP → ↑−dP/dt

Time constant of relaxation (τ)

$$\tau = -1/A$$

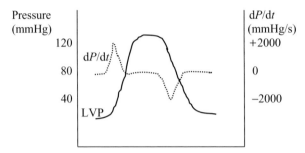

Fig. 4.3

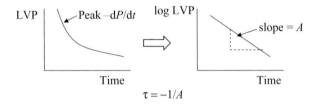

Fig. 4.4

$= 25\text{–}40$ ms

↓LVP during IVRT $=$ exponential decay (Fig. 4.4)

Chamber stiffness

Passive property of myocardium

Reciprocal of compliance, i.e. dP/dV

Affected by:

    LV volume

    LV mass

    RV pressure

    pericardial pressure

    pleural pressure

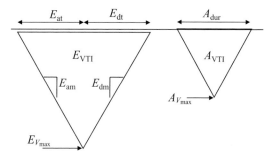

Fig. 4.5

Diastolic dysfunction

IVRT
Impaired relaxation → ↑IVRT > 90 ms
Restrictive pathology → ↓IVRT < 70 ms

Transmitral flow (Fig. 4.5)
LV filling depends on:
(1) LAP:LVP gradient
    LAP – LA Cn/LA contractility
    LVP – LV Cn/LV relaxation/LVESV
(2) MV area
Impaired relaxation:
    $\downarrow E_{V_{max}}/\uparrow A_{V_{max}}$
    $\downarrow E_{VTI}/\uparrow A_{VTI}$
    $\downarrow E_{am}/\uparrow E_{at}$
    $\downarrow E_{dm}/\uparrow E_{dt}$
    $\downarrow E/A/\downarrow E_{VTI}/A_{VTI}$
Restrictive pathology:
    $\uparrow E_{V_{max}}/\downarrow A_{V_{max}}$
    $\uparrow E_{VTI}/\downarrow A_{VTI}$
    $\uparrow E_{dm}/\downarrow E_{dt}$
    $\uparrow E/A$

Pulmonary vein flow

Impaired relaxation $\rightarrow \uparrow PV_S / \downarrow PV_D$

$\rightarrow \uparrow PV_A$ duration

Restrictive pathology $\rightarrow \downarrow PV_S / \uparrow PV_D$

Physiological effects

(1) Respiration: inspiration causes $\uparrow$TTF $E_{V_{max}} / \downarrow$TMF $E_{V_{max}}$

(2) Heart rate:

$\uparrow$HR causes $\downarrow E_{V_{max}} / \uparrow A_{V_{max}}$

$\uparrow\uparrow$HR causes A on E (A incorporated into E)

(3) Age:

$\uparrow$age causes $\downarrow E_{V_{max}} / \uparrow A_{V_{max}}$

$\uparrow$IVRT

$\uparrow E_{dt}$

(4) AV interval:

prolonged PR interval delays LV contraction

$\rightarrow$ delays E wave

$\rightarrow E$ and A fuse

Pathological states

(1) LV hypertrophy: $\downarrow E/A$

(2) Ischaemia: $\downarrow E/A$

$\uparrow E_{dt}$

(3) RVP: pulmonary $\uparrow$BP $\rightarrow \downarrow E/A$ and $\uparrow$IVRT

volume overload $\rightarrow \uparrow E/A$ and IVRT$\leftrightarrow$

(4) Tamponade: exaggerated TTF $\uparrow E_{V_{max}}$ on inspiration

(5) Pericardial constriction: $\uparrow$IVRT$/ \downarrow E_{V_{max}}$ on inspiration

Table 4.1 Diastolic dysfunction summary

	Normal	Impaired relaxation	Pseudo-normal	Restrictive pathology
DT (ms)	160–240	>240	160–200	<160
IVRT (ms)	70–90	>90	>90	<70
E/A	1–2	<1	1–1.5	>2
A_{dur}/PV_{Adur}	$A>PV_A$	$A>PV_A$	$A<PV_A$	$A<<PV_A$
PV_S/PV_D	$PV_S>PV_D$	$PV_S>>PV_D$	$PV_S<PV_D$	$PV_S<<PV_D$
E_{VTI}/A_{VTI}	$E>A$	$E<A$	$E>A$	$E>>A$
Valsalva E: A	↓↓	↓↓	↓↑	↓↓

Summary of diastolic dysfunction (Table 4.1)

RV function

Normal RV function

RV = triangular/crescent-shaped
Contains muscle ridges = trabeculae carneae
Moderator band: large muscle bundle from low IVS to ant RV wall

Velocity of RV ejection:
  ↑ gradually
  peaks later than LV
  persists longer than LV

RV volume determined by Simpson's method

RV dysfunction

Volume overload
Dilated RV
Flattening of IVS (moves to left)

Pressure overload

(1) Chronic:

      e.g. pulmonary hypertension

      RV hypertrophy (RV free wall thickness > 5 mm)

      progresses to RV dilatation/free wall hypokinesia

(2) Acute:

      e.g. PE

      RV can compensate to PAP < 40 mmHg

      RV dilatation with TR

      RV free wall hypokinesia

      IVS flattening in diastole

      RA/IVC dilatation

Multiple choice questions

1. For an adult female, left ventricular hypertrophy is defined as a left ventricular mass of greater than

    A 12 mg/m^2

    B 120 mg/m^2

    C 12 g/m^2

    D 120 g/m^2

    E 1.2 kg/m^2

2. If the left ventricular internal diameter in systole is 30 mm and the left ventricular internal diameter in diastole is 45 mm, the fractional shortening is approximately

    A 15%

    B 25%

    C 33%

    D 50%

    E 66%

3. In mitral regurgitation

    A ejection fraction is preserved until late in the disease

B there is commonly left ventricular concentric hypertrophy

C prognosis is poor if fractional shortening is less than 42%

D there is a reduction in left ventricular end diastolic volume

E there is a reduction in left ventricular end systolic volume

4. The following statements regarding segmental left ventricular function are all true except

A regional wall motion abnormality occurs 5–10 beats after coronary occlusion

B right coronary artery supplies the inferior wall

C pacing can cause a regional wall motion abnormality

D left circumflex coronary artery supplies the lateral wall

E post-myocardial infarction scarring often causes wall thickening greater than 9 mm

5. A normal isovolumic relaxation time is

A 7–9 µs

B 70–90 µs

C 0.7–0.9 ms

D 7–9 ms

E 70–90 ms

6. Isovolumic relaxation

A commences when the mitral valve closes

B involves a 35% reduction in left ventricular volume

C terminates when left atrial pressure exceeds left ventricular pressure

D terminates when the mitral valve closes

E commences when the aortic valve opens

7. Chamber stiffness is affected by all of the following except

A left ventricle volume

B right ventricle pressure

C pericardial pressure

D pleural pressure

E ascending aortic compliance

8. Regarding impaired relaxation, there is
   A an increase in *E* wave maximum velocity
   B a decrease in *A* wave maximum velocity
   C an increase in the *E/A* ratio
   D an increase in pulmonary vein flow *A* wave duration
   E an increase in pulmonary vein flow *D* wave velocity

9. Regarding transmitral flow
   A impaired relaxation causes shortening of the *E* wave acceleration time
   B restrictive pathology causes an increase in *E* wave deceleration time
   C inspiration causes increased *E* wave velocity
   D increasing heart rate causes reduced *E/A* ratio
   E restrictive pathology causes increased *A* wave velocity

10. Regarding restrictive pathology
    A isovolumic relaxation time is often greater than 90 ms
    B deceleration time is usually less than 160 ms
    C *E/A* ratio is greatly reduced
    D transmitral *A* wave duration greatly exceeds pulmonary vein flow *A* wave duration
    E pulmonary vein flow *S* wave velocity greatly exceeds *D* wave velocity

11. Increasing age causes
    A increase in isovolumic relaxation time
    B increase in *E* wave maximum velocity
    C decrease in *E* wave deceleration time
    D decrease in *A* wave maximum velocity
    E increase in *E/A* ratio

12. The following statements about the right ventricle are all true except
    A the normal right ventricle is crescent shaped
    B it contains muscle ridges called trabeculae carneae
    C in right ventricular hypertrophy the free wall is usually thicker than 15 mm
    D its volume can be determined using Simpson's method
    E acute pulmonary embolism can cause right ventricular free wall hypokinesia

5

Cardiomyopathies

Hypertrophic obstructive cardiomyopathy

Definition and epidemiology

Unexplained hypertrophy of non-dilated LV
Prevalence ~ 1–2% of population
Familial autosomal dominant ≈ 55%
Sporadic ≈ 45%

Features

Asymmetric septal hypertrophy

(1) Type I: anteroseptal
(2) Type II: panseptal
(3) Type III: extensive, sparing only posterior wall
(4) Type IV: apico-septal

IVS: posterior wall thickness ratio > 1.3:1

Systolic anterior motion (SAM) of anterior MV leaflet (AMVL)

= functional subaortic stenosis
Common with large, redundant AMVL
Anterior motion of antero-lateral papillary muscle
Venturi effect causes suction of AMVL into LVOT
LVOT PG > 36 mmHg (velocity > 3 m/s)
CW Doppler → 'dagger-shaped' pattern with late peaking

Mitral regurgitation

Magnitude of MR greatest in mid- to late-systole

Early AV closure

Mid-systolic AV closure

Dilated cardiomyopathy

Definition

Four-chamber enlargement with impaired RV and LV
systolic function

Aetiology

Idiopathic
IHD
Post-partum
Post-CPB
Toxins – alcohol, cobalt, adriamycin, snake bites
Metabolic – acromegaly, thiamine, and selenium deficiency
Infection – post-viral, Chagas' disease
Inherited – Duchenne's muscular dystrophy, SC anaemia
Systemic disease – haemoachromatosis: Fe deposition within myocytes
  in epicardial region → fibrosis

Features

Four-chamber dilatation
RV and LV systolic dysfunction +/− diastolic
  dysfunction
Normal wall thickness
Increased LV mass

LV inflow directed postero-laterally
May have predominantly RV dilatation (Coxsackie B infection)

Restrictive cardiomyopathy

Causes

Idiopathic
Amyloid
Sarcoid
Storage diseases
Carcinoid
Endocardial fibroelastosis
Endomyocardial fibrosis

Features

Biatrial dilatation
Normal ventricular size and systolic function
Restriction to RV and LV filling
Echo-dense RV and LV walls

Amyloidosis

Deposition of abnormal proteins between myocardial fibres, in
    PMs, in conductive tissue and in pericardium
Increased RV and LV wall thickness
'Speckled'/granular appearance
RV/LV size and systolic function normal
Biatrial dilatation
Diffuse valvular thickening (MV and TV)
Small/moderate effusion

Sarcoidosis

Non-caseating granulomas

Affects LV free wall, IVS (conduction tissue), PMs causing MR and LV
dilatation with RWMA

Storage diseases

Accumulation of abnormal metabolites

(1) Glycogen (Pompe's/Cori's): LVH +/− SAM
(2) Lipid (Fabry's) ≡ amyloidosis
(3) Mucopolysaccharide (Hurler's, Sanfilipo etc.): MV thickening

Carcinoid

Malignant tumour with hepatic metastases

Endocardial injury due to hormones (serotonin, kinins)

RA wall/TV/PV thickening

Usually TR + PS

Primary bronchogenic tumour can cause left-sided lesions

Endocardial fibroelastosis

Diffuse endocardial hyperplasia

Increased chamber size and wall thickness

AV/MV fibrosis

Endomyocardial fibrosis (Loeffler's endocarditis)

Assoc. with:
idiopathic hypereosinophilic syndrome, acquired
hypereosinophilia

Fibrosis affecting :
MV/TV   } MR/MS
subvalvular apparatus } TR/TS
apex

Increased risk of thrombus formation

Preserved LV systolic function

Multiple choice questions

1. Regarding hypertrophic obstructive cardiomyopathy
  A the prevalence is 0.1%
  B type II septal hypertrophy is limited to the apex
  C more than 65% of cases are sporadic
  D type III septal hypertrophy is limited to the posterior wall
  E the interventricular septum : posterior wall thickness ratio is usually greater than 1.3

2. Systolic anterior motion of the anterior mitral valve leaflet
  A creates a functional sub-aortic stenosis
  B is common with a small, redundant anterior leaflet
  C is associated with posterior motion of the antero-lateral papillary muscle
  D is associated with a fall in the pressure gradient across the left ventricular outflow tract
  E creates a 'dagger-shaped' pattern with early peaking on application of continuous wave Doppler

3. The following statements about dilated cardiomyopathy are all true except
  A it may be caused by cobalt toxicity
  B there is an increase in left ventricular mass
  C left ventricular inflow is directed antero-laterally
  D left ventricular wall thickness is normal
  E left ventricular diastolic dysfunction may occur

4. Features typical of restrictive cardiomyopathy include
  A right ventricular dilatation in amyloidosis
  B aortic and mitral valve fibrosis in endocardial fibroelastosis
  C reduced left atrial size in sarcoidosis
  D reduced left ventricular systolic function in endomyocardial fibrosis
  E echolucent ventricular walls in amyloidosis

6

Valvular heart disease

Mitral valve

Mitral stenosis

Aetiology
Rheumatic
Degenerative calcification
Congenital
Vegetations
Parachute MV (chordae attached to single PM)
Infiltrative (fibrosis, amyloid)
Ergot, hypereosinophilia, non-valvular (myxoma, thrombus)

Features
M Mode
  ↓E-F slope of AMVL
  Anterior motion of PMVL
2-D
  Reduced leaflet motion
  Leaflet thickening
  Reduced orifice size
  AMVL 'hockey stick' appearance
  'diastolic doming' – body of leaflets more pliable and receive some of
    blood flowing from LA to LV
  LA – enlarged/'smoke'/thrombus/AF
  LAA – 'smoke'/thrombus/reduced Doppler velocities
  LV – small/underfilled
  Signs of pulmonary hypertension (RA/RV enlarged)

Table 6.1 Assessment of mitral stenosis by mean pressure gradient (MG) and mitral valve area (MVA)

Severity	MG (mmHg)	MVA (cm^2)
Normal	0	4–6
Mild	<6	2–4
Moderate	6–12	1–2
Severe	> 12	<1

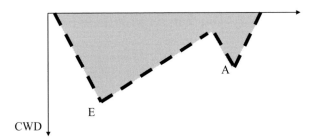

Fig. 6.1

Rheumatic MS
Calcification of MV and subvalvular apparatus
Fusion of commissures and chordae
'Fish-mouth' MV orifice

Assessment of MS severity

(1) Planimetry:
      trace 'fish-mouth' in transgastric basal SAX view
      affected by plane and gain
      TOE underestimates degree of MS

(2) Transvalvular gradient: uses modified Bernoulli equation

$$P = 4V^2$$

      Use mean pressure gradient (MG) (Table 6.1)
      Trace around *E* and *A* waves (Fig. 6.1)
      Underestimates degree of MS if AI present

Three-chamber   Two-chamber

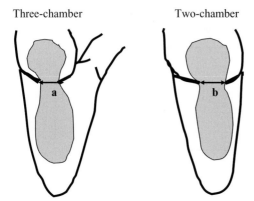

Fig. 6.2

(3) Continuity equation:

$$\text{Flow} = \text{Velocity} \times \text{Area}$$
$$V_1 A_1 = V_2 A_2$$
$$A_2 = V_1 A_1 / V_2$$
$$\text{MVA} = V_{\text{LVOT}} \times A_{\text{LVOT}} / V_{\text{MV}}$$
$$\text{MVA} = \text{VTI}_{\text{LVOT}} \times A_{\text{LVOT}} / \text{VTI}_{\text{MV}}$$

Inaccurate with AI (affects VTI_{LVOT})

(4) Colour flow Doppler area (Fig. 6.2)

$$\text{MVA} = (\pi/4)\,(ab)$$
$$\text{MVA} = 0.785\,(ab)$$

(5) Pressure half time (PHT) (Fig. 6.3)
Time taken for pressure to fall by $^1/_2$
Inaccurate with AI: AI $\rightarrow$ $\downarrow$PHT $\rightarrow$ overestimates MVA

$$\text{MVA} = 220/\text{PHT}$$

(6) Depressurization time (DepT) (Fig. 6.3)

$$\text{MVA} = 750/\text{DepT}$$

(7) Proximal isovelocity surface area (PISA). Flow converges uniformly and radially towards a small orifice, creating concentric isovelocity layers

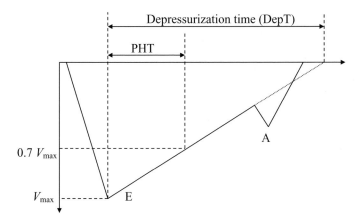

Fig. 6.3

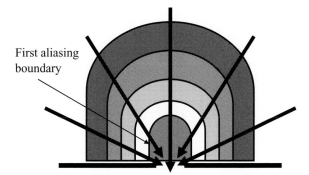

Fig. 6.4

When orifice is very small compared to region of acceleration the isovelocity surfaces are hemispheric (Fig. 6.4)

Flow through isovelocity surface = velocity × area

Conservation of mass : flow at each surface = orifice flow

If orifice flow known, orifice area calculated: area = flow/velocity

At first aliasing boundary: flow = area $(2\pi r^2)$ × V_{alias}

Correction for funnel-shaped inflow angle α

$$MVA = 2\pi r^2 \times \alpha/180 \times V_{alias}/V_{max}$$
$$MVA = 6.28r^2 \times \alpha/180 \times V_{alias}/V_{max}$$

(8) Gorlin formula: used in cardiac catheter lab

$$MVA = CO/[(DFT \times HR)(44 \times C \times \sqrt{MG})]$$

CO = cardiac output
DFT = diastolic filling time
HR = heart rate
C = orifice constant (for MV = 0.85)
MG = mean gradient

$$MVA = CO/[(DFT \times HR)(37.5\sqrt{MG})]$$

Mitral regurgitation

Aetiology

(1) Congenital
   Cleft MV
   Double-orifice MV
   Mitral arcade
(2) Acquired
   Rheumatic
   Ischaemic
   MV prolapse
   PM dysfunction/rupture
   Chordal dysfunction/rupture
   Vegetation
(3) Other
   MV aneurysm
   Annular calcification
   Fibrosis
   Tumours

Carpentier classification

I: normal leaflet motion:
   dilated annulus
   leaflet perforation

II: excessive leaflet motion:
  myxomatous disease
  PM/chordal rupture
  MV prolapse
  flail
III: restricted leaflet motion:
  rheumatic disease
  chordal tethering (ischaemia)

Assessment of MR severity

  (1) Jet length
  Trivial <1.5 cm
  Mild 1.5–3 cm
  Moderate 3–4.5 cm
  Severe >4.5 cm
  (2) Jet length/LA length
  Trivial <25%
  Mild 25–50%
  Moderate 50–75%
  Severe >75%
  (3) Jet area
  Trivial <1.5 cm^2
  Mild 1.5–4 cm^2
  Moderate 4–7 cm^2
  Severe >7 cm^2
  (4) Jet area/LA area
  Mild <20%
  Moderate 20–40%
  Severe >40%
  (5) Qualitative
  Signal strength with CW Doppler
  i.e. large volume MR gives strong CW signal
  (6) Regurgitant volume (RV)
  Difference between MV diastolic flow and AV systolic flow,
    assuming no AI

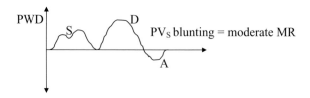

PV$_S$ blunting = moderate MR

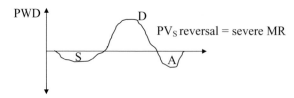

PV$_S$ reversal = severe MR

Fig. 6.5

Severe >60 ml

$$RV = MV\,vol - LVOT\,vol$$
$$RV = (Area_{MV} \times VTI_{MV}) - (Area_{LVOT} \times VTI_{LVOT})$$

(7) Regurgitant fraction
   Trivial <20%
   Mild 20–30%
   Moderate 30–50%
   Severe >50%

(8) Effective regurgitant orifice (ERO): from PISA
   Mild <0.2 cm^2
   Moderate 0.2–0.4 cm^2
   Severe >0.4 cm^2

$$ERO = 6.28r^2 \times V_{alias} / V_{MR}$$

(9) Pulmonary venous flow (Fig. 6.5)
   Moderate PV$_S$ blunting
   Severe PV$_S$ reversal

(10) Vena contracta
   Narrowest portion of jet downstream from orifice
   >0.5 cm ≡ ERO >0.4 cm^2

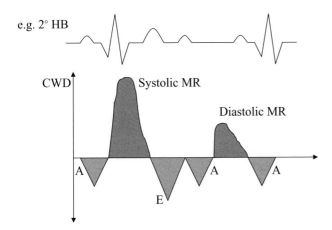

Fig. 6.6

Diastolic MR
Retrograde flow from LV to LA during diastole (Fig. 6.6)
Causes include AV block, atrial flutter, severe AI, high LVEDP

Mitral valve prolapse
Displacement of MV leaflet >3 mm above level of annulus
Occurs mid/end systole as annulus moves towards apex
    Bilateral leaflet prolapse: 75–90%
    Posterior leaflet prolapse: 10–20%
    Anterior leaflet prolapse: 3–5%

Associated with infective endocarditis, MR, sudden death from
    ventricular arrhythmias

Aortic valve

Aortic stenosis

Aetiology
(1) Congenital
    Uni-/bi-/quadricuspid valve

(2) Acquired

    Rheumatic

    Degenerative calcification

    Amyloid

Features
Thick, immobile, calcified AV leaflets

Commissural fusion (rheumatic)

'Doming' of AV leaflets

Reduced AV opening

Associated LVH $+/-$ dilated aortic root

Assessment of AS severity
(1) Planimetry: severe AS suggested if AV area <0.7 cm^2

(2) Continuity equation

$$AVA = A_{LVOT} \times VTI_{LVOT} / VTI_{AV}$$
$$AVA = A_{LVOT} \times V_{LVOT} / V_{AV}$$

(3) Gorlin formula

$$AVA = CO/HR \times ET \times 44\sqrt{MG}$$

    CO $=$ Cardiac output

    HR $=$ Heart rate

    ET $=$ Ejection time

    MG $=$ Mean gradient

(4) Doppler pressure gradients: normal $V_{max} <1.5$ m/s (Table 6.2)

Peak PG vs. 'Peak-to-peak' PG (Fig. 6.7)
$P_1 =$ peak PG by Doppler

Instantaneous

Maximum difference between aorta and LV pressures during systole at
one instant in time

$P_2 =$ 'peak-to-peak' pressure in cardiac catheter lab

Table 6.2 Assessment of aortic stenosis by peak pressure gradient (PG), mean PG and aortic valve area (AVA)

	Peak PG (mmHg)	Mean PG (mmHg)	AVA (cm²)
Normal	–	–	2–4.5
Mild	<40	<20	1–2
Moderate	40–80	20–50	0.7–1.0
Severe	>80	>50	<0.7

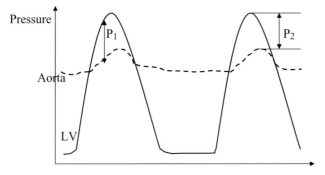

Fig. 6.7

Non-simultaneous difference between peak aortic and peak LV
    pressures
$P_1 > P_2$
Mean PG measured with Doppler and cardiac catheter usually equal

Aortic insufficiency

Aetiology
(1) Congenital
        Uni-/bi-/quadricuspid valve
(2) Acquired
    (a) Leaflet pathology:
        Degeneration
        Rheumatic

Infective endocarditis

Trauma

(b) Annulus pathology:

Infection (syphilis)

Thoracic aortic aneurysm

Ascending aortic dissection

Features

Premature closure of MV

Poor coaptation of AV leaflets

Dilated aortic root

Assessment of AI severity

(1) Jet length (inaccurate)

Mild <2 cm

Moderate 2 cm papillary muscles

Severe beyond papillary muscles

(2) Perry index $=$ jet height/LVOT diameter

Mild <25%

Moderate 25–60%

Severe >60%

(3) Regurgitant fraction/volume

$RF = (Vol_{AI}/Vol_{LVOT}) \times 100$

Mild <30%

Moderate 30–50%

Severe >50%

Regurgitant volume > 60 ml $=$ severe AI

(4) Pressure half-time (PHT)

Mild >550 ms

Moderate 300–550 ms

Severe <300 ms

(5) Flow reversal

Mild ascending aorta

Moderate descending thoracic aorta

Severe abdominal aorta

Table 6.3 Assessment of aortic incompetence using Perry index, pressure half-time (PHT), regurgitant fraction (RF) and aortic flow reversal (AoFR)

	Perry index (%)	PHT (ms)	RF (%)	AoFR
Mild	<25	>550	<30	Ascending aorta
Moderate	25–60	300–550	30–50	Desc. thor. aorta
Severe	>60	<300	>50	Abdominal aorta

Summary of AI assessment (Table 6.3)

Tricuspid valve

Tricuspid stenosis

Aetiology
(1) Congenital

   TV atresia associated with RV hypoplasia
(2) Acquired

   Rheumatic

   Carcinoid

   Endocardial fibroelastosis

   Endomyocardial fibrosis

Features
Scarred, thickened leaflets/chordae

Commissural fusion (rheumatic)

Reduced leaflet opening

'Doming' of ant. leaflet (rheumatic)

Assessment of TS severity
(1) Planimetry: inaccurate due to position of TV attachments
(2) Doppler pressure gradient (Table 6.4)
(3) Continuity equation:

$$TVA = MVA \times VTI_{MV}/VTI_{TV}$$

Inaccurate with TR

Table 6.4 Assessment of tricuspid stenosis by mean pressure gradient (PG)

	Mean PG (mmHg)
Mild	<3
Moderate	3–6
Severe	>6

(4) Pressure half-time (PHT):

$$TVA = 190/PHT$$

Tricuspid regurgitation

Mild–moderate TR common in normal population
↑TR with age
↑TR with physical fitness

Aetiology
(1) Congenital
      TV dysplasia
      Ebstein's anomaly
(2) Acquired
      Rheumatic
      Annular dilatation due to RV dilatation
      TV prolapse
      Carcinoid
      Infective endocarditis
      Tumours
      Trauma

Features
Ebstein's
  – apical attachment of TV leaflets (usually septal leaflet)
  – atrialization of RV
  – dilated RA/small RV
  – septal TVL attaches to IVS >8 mm/m^2 (BSA) below anterior MVL

RV dilatation/pulmonary ↑BP (annular dilatation)

RA/IVC dilatation

TV prolapse assoc. with MV prolapse/Marfan's syndrome

Infective endocarditis assoc. with IV drug use/alcoholism

Thick, short TV leaflets with reduced motion (carcinoid)

Assessment of TR severity

(1) Jet length

Trivial <1.5 cm

Mild 1.5–3 cm

Moderate 3–4.5 cm

Severe >4.5 cm

(2) Jet area

Trivial <2 cm^2

Mild 2–4 cm^2

Moderate 4–10 cm^2

Severe > 10 cm^2

(3) Jet length/RA length

Mild <33%

Moderate 33–66%

Severe >66%

(4) Jet area/RA area

Mild < 33%

Moderate 33–66%

Severe > 66%

(5) Systolic flow reversal in IVC/hepatic vein = severe TR

Pulmonary valve

Pulmonary stenosis

Aetiology

(1) Congenital

Uni-/bi-/quadricuspid valve

Fallot's tetralogy

Table 6.5 Assessment of pulmonary insufficiency by regurgitant fraction (RF)

	RF (%)
Mild	<40
Moderate	40–60
Severe	>60

(2) Acquired
     Carcinoid
     Rheumatic

Features
Thickened leaflets
'Doming' of leaflets
$\uparrow V_{max} > 1$ m/s

Pulmonary insufficiency

Aetiology
(1) Congenital
     Uni-/bi-/quadricuspid valve
(2) Acquired
     Carcinoid
     Infective endocarditis

Assessment of PI severity
(1) Regurgitant fraction (Table 6.5)

Valve surgery

Mitral valve repair

Repair:
   reduced morbidity and mortality

better durability
preserves tensor apparatus
avoids anticoagulation

BUT: 6–8% inadequate

Better for:
   PMVL
   annular dilatation
   no calcification

(1) Carpentier I (normal leaflet motion)
Ring annuloplasty

(2) Carpentier II (↑leaflet motion)
Quadrangular resection of PMVL (usually P2)
Shortening of AMVL chordae
Transposition of PMVL chordae to AMVL
Secondary chordae transposition from AMVL body to leaflet tips
Partial resection of AMVL + ring annuloplasty

(3) Carpentier III (↓leaflet motion)
Commissurotomy
Resection of secondary chordae/fenestration of primary chordae
Resection of fused chordae
Balloon valvuloplasty

Valve replacement

Homografts
From cadaveric human hearts/cryopreserved

(1) Unstented:
      usually AV
      avoids anticoagulation
      good durability

(2) Stented:
    usually MV
    duration ~ 5 yrs

Bioprostheses

(1) Porcine:
    Hancock/Carpentier–Edwards
    premounted porcine AV
    leaflet degeneration/calcification
    duration ~ 5–10 yrs
(2) Bovine:
    Ionescu–Shiley
    bovine pericardium
    calcification/abrasions → stenosis and regurgitation
    duration ~ 5–10 yrs

Mechanical valves

(1) Ball-and-cage:
    Starr–Edwards
    Double cage with silastic ball
    Haemolysis occurs in AV position
    Duration ~ 20 yrs
(2) Single tilting disc:
    Bjork–Shiley/Medtronics
    Single-hinged mobile disc
    Eccentric attachment
    Good durability
(3) Bileaflet tilting disc:
    St Jude
    Equal-sized semicircular leaflets with midline hinge

Normal valve replacement gradients (Table 6.6)

Table 6.6a Mean pressure gradients (PG) measured across different mitral valve replacements (MVR)

MVR	Mean PG (mmHg)
Carpentier–Edwards	6.5 +/− 2.1
Hancock	4.3 +/− 2.1
Starr–Edwards	4.5 +/− 2.4
St Jude	3.5 +/− 1.3
Bjork–Shiley	2.9 +/− 1.6

Table 6.6b Mean and peak pressure gradients (PG) measured across different aortic valve replacements (AVR)

AVR	Mean PG (mmHg)	Peak PG (mmHg)
Carpentier–Edwards	12 +/− 6	23 +/− 8
Hancock	11 + /− 2	22 +/− 10
Starr–Edwards	24 +/− 4	39 +/− 12
Bjork–Shiley	14 +/− 5	24 +/− 9
St Jude	13 +/− 6	26 +/− 5

Multiple choice questions

1. Typical features of mitral stenosis include all of the following except
   A dilated left ventricle
   B thrombus in the left atrial appendage
   C commissural fusion
   D atrial fibrillation
   E 'hockey stick' appearance of the anterior leaflet
2. Regarding the assessment of mitral stenosis severity, the following statement is correct
   A pressure half-time is reduced with aortic incompetence

    B transvalvular gradient overestimates the degree of mitral stenosis in the presence of aortic incompetence

    C the continuity equation is accurate in the presence of aortic incompetence

    D planimetry often overestimates the degree of mitral stenosis

    E a depressurization time of 550 ms equates to severe mitral stenosis

3. Mitral regurgitation

    A cannot be caused by myocardial ischaemia

    B is classified as severe if the effective regurgitant orifice is greater than 0.4 cm^2

    C is classified as severe if the regurgitant volume is greater than 40 ml

    D due to excessive leaflet motion is classified as Carpentier I

    E due to myxomatous disease is usually classified as Carpentier III

4. In moderate mitral regurgitation

    A the jet length is typically 1–2 cm

    B the jet area is 4–7 cm^2

    C the regurgitant fraction is 50–75%

    D there is reversal of pulmonary vein flow *S* wave

    E the vena contracta is 0.5–0.75 cm

5. Causes of aortic stenosis include all of the following except

    A congenital unicuspid valve

    B congenital bicuspid valve

    C degenerative calcification

    D amyloidosis

    E myocardial ischaemia

6. A mean pressure gradient of 40 mmHg across the aortic valve equates to

    A aortic valve area of 2–4.5 cm^2

    B mild aortic stenosis

    C moderate aortic stenosis

    D a peak pressure gradient of 100 mmHg

    E aortic valve area of 4–6 cm^2

7. Features of mild aortic valve incompetence include

    A Perry index greater than 60%

    B regurgitant fraction greater than 60%

C regurgitant volume greater than 60 ml

D pressure half-time greater than 600 ms

E diastolic flow reversal in the abdominal aorta

8. **In aortic incompetence, a Perry index of 50% is consistent with**

   A pressure half-time of 550 ms

   B regurgitant fraction of 25%

   C diastolic flow reversal in the descending thoracic aorta

   D diastolic flow reversal in the abdominal aorta

   E pressure half-time of 750 ms

9. **In the assessment of tricuspid stenosis severity**

   A planimetry is the most accurate method

   B mean pressure gradient of 9 mmHg is severe stenosis

   C the continuity equation is accurate in the presence of tricuspid regurgitation

   D pressure half-time of 220 ms is mild stenosis

   E pressure half-time of 110 ms gives an approximate tricuspid valve area of 2.2 cm^2

10. **The following statements regarding tricuspid regurgitation are all true except**

    A Ebstein's anomaly results in a small right atrium with a dilated right ventricle

    B carcinoid disease is a cause

    C a jet length of 7 cm is considered to be severe

    D a jet area of 11 cm^2 is severe

    E mild regurgitation is common in the normal population

11. **The maximum velocity across a normal pulmonary valve is**

    A 1–2 cm/s

    B 6–9 cm/s

    C 10–20 cm/s

    D 60–90 cm/s

    E 1–1.2 m/s

12. **Regarding heart valve surgery**

    A St Jude valve is an example of a bileaflet tilting disc

B ring annuloplasty is usually not suitable for Carpentier I mitral regurgitation

C the mean pressure gradient across a Hancock mitral valve replacement is approximately 11–12 mmHg

D the advantage of valve replacement is avoidance of anticoagulation treatment

E commissurotomy is suitable for Carpentier II mitral regurgitation

7

Cardiac masses

Tumours

Primary tumours

Myxoma

A myxoid matrix of acid mucopolysaccharide and polygonal cells

Benign
25% of all primary cardiac tumours
75% in LA/20% in RA/5% other sites in heart
LA myxomas: 90% on IAS (fossa ovalis)
Usually present between 30 and 60 years of age
May be part of a syndrome (Carney's complex)
Homogenous echo appearance
May contain calcium, haemorrhage or secondary
    infection
Soft, friable, gelatinous, and pedunculated

Features:
    disruption of MV function
    emboli
    systemic symptoms (fever, malaise)

Lipoma

Occur throughout the heart
Subepicardial: large, smooth, and pedunculated
Subendocardial: small and sessile
Less mobile/more echodense than myxomas

May cause arrhythmias/conduction defects
May present with pericardial effusion

Papillary fibroelastoma
Small (usually < 1 cm)
Attached to valve surfaces/supporting valvular apparatus
Round/oval tumour with well-demarcated border
Homogeneous texture
May cause systemic embolization

Rhabdomyoma
Common paediatric primary tumour
Assoc. with tuberous sclerosis
90% multiple/nodular masses
Associated with outflow tract obstruction
May resolve spontaneously

Fibroma
Solitary
Occur in LV/RV myocardium
Firm with central calcification
May appear as localized irregular myocardial hypertrophy
May be mistaken as thrombus at the apex of the heart
Cause dysrhythmias and congestive cardiac failure

Haemangioma
Solitary and small
Occur in RV/IVS/AV node
Cause complete heart block

Cysts
Mesotheliomas: primary malignant tumour of pericardium
Teratomas: intrapericardial or intracardiac
Benign cysts: fluid-filled recesses of parietal pericardium
Echinococcal cyst: secondary to echinococcosis

Malignant tumours

25% of all primary cardiac tumours are malignant

Angiosarcomas

Rhabdomyosarcomas

Lymphosarcomas

Secondary tumours

Cardiac metastases reported in up to 20% of patients with malignant tumours.

Metastases by

(1) direct extension
(2) lymphatic spread (carcinoma)
(3) haematogenous spread (melanoma/sarcoma)

Common primary malignancy metastasizing to the heart include

(1) lung
(2) breast
(3) melanoma
(4) leukaemia
(5) lymphoma
(6) ovary
(7) oesophagus
(8) kidney

Most common spread to heart via IVC includes

(1) renal cell carcinoma
(2) Wilms' tumour (paediatric)
(3) uterine leiomyosarcoma
(4) hepatoma

Carcinoid syndrome

Patient with carcinoid tumour of ileum with hepatic metastases

Right-sided heart lesions

Left-sided lesions with bronchial carcinoid/ASD/PFO
Endocardial thickening causing fixation of TV and PV
TR universal finding, usually with PS

Thrombus

Found in setting of
   Blood stasis
   AF
   Reduced CO states
   MV disease
   Prosthetic MV
   Post-MI
   RWMA

Features
Round/oval masses
'Speckled' with ↑echodensity compared to LA/LV wall
Interrupts normal endocardial contour
Posterior and lateral walls of LA/LAA
Apex of LV
Associated with 'smoke' in LA

Effects
Mechanical disruption of valve function
Causes emboli

Pseudomasses

Trabeculations
Muscle bundles on endocardial surfaces
More common in RA/RV than LA/LV

Accentuated by RVH

May occur in LAA

False tendons

Fine filamentous structures in LV

No clinical significance

Pectinate muscles

Parallel ridges across anterior endocardium of LA (LAA) and RA

No clinical significance

Moderator band

Prominent muscle band in apical third of RV

Involved with conduction system

Confused with thrombus/tumour

Lipomatous hypertrophy of IAS

Lipomatous thickening of IAS > 1 cm

Benign

'Dumb-bell' appearance of IAS

Lack of involvement of fossa ovalis

Eustachian valve

= Remnant of valve of sinus venosus

Occurs in 25% of individuals

At junction of IVC and RA

Elongated, membranous undulating structure

Chiari network

? Remnant of sinus venosus derived structures

Mobile, filamentous, thin structure in RA

Highly mobile/random movement in RA

? Associated with PFO/IAS aneurysm

Crista terminalis
= Remnant of valve of sinus venosus
At junction of SVC and RA

Thebesian valve
Thin piece of tissue guarding coronary sinus
May inhibit retrograde coronary sinus cannulation

Warfarin ridge
Atrial tissue separating LAA from LUPV

Vegetations

TTE sensitivity ~ 80%
TOE sensitivity ~ 95% (reduced with prosthetic valves)

Features
Classic triad
   changing murmur
   fever
   positive blood cultures
Variable appearance
   discrete sessile mass
   pedunculated friable clump
   elongated strand
Occur on low pressure side of valves
Usually at leaflet tips
Right-sided vegetations usually larger than left-sided
Fungal vegetations larger than bacterial
Chronic, healed vegetation = fibrotic and echodense

Multiple choice questions

1. Atrial myxomas
   A comprise 75% of all primary cardiac tumours
   B usually arise from the appendage in the left atrium
   C are usually malignant
   D cause systemic symptoms of fever and malaise
   E occur in the right atrium in 5% of cases
2. Features of cardiac thrombus include all of the following except
   A association with 'smoke' in the left atrium
   B association with reduced cardiac output states
   C 'speckled' oval mass in the left atrial appendage
   D reduced echodensity compared to the ventricular wall
   E mechanical disruption of valve function
3. The following statements regarding cardiac pseudomasses are all true
   except
   A false tendons occur in the left ventricle
   B trabeculations are muscle bundles on epicardial surfaces
   C the Eustachian valve is the embryological remnant of the valve of the
   sinus venosus
   D the crista terminalis occurs at the junction of the right atrium and the
   superior vena cava
   E a thebesian valve may inhibit retrograde coronary sinus cannulation
4. Regarding cardiac vegetations
   A transthoracic echocardiography is more sensitive than
   transoesophageal echocardiography for diagnosis
   B transoesophageal echocardiogram sensitivity is increased in the
   presence of prosthetic heart valves
   C they usually occur on the high pressure side of valves
   D right-sided vegetations are usually larger than left-sided
   E bacterial vegetations are usually larger than fungal ones

8

Congenital heart disease

Valve defects

Mitral valve

Parachute MV
Normal leaflets attach to single, large papillary muscle
Reduced leaflet motion → MS

Cleft mitral valve
'Clefts' in ant MV leaflet
Accessory chordae attach to cleft margins, holding leaflets anteriorly
during systole → MR

Mitral arcade
Fibrous bridge between papillary muscles with poor commissural
development
Arcade prevents closure of AMVL → MR

Aortic valve

Unicuspid
Acommissural with central orifice
Commissural with eccentric orifice → AS

Bicuspid
Most common congenital cardiac defect (1–2% of population)
AS + AI

Common site for bacterial endocarditis
Associated with coarctation/PDA/ascending aortic aneurysm

Quadricuspid

AI
Associated with truncus arteriosus

Tricuspid valve

Atresia

Large RA/hypoplastic RV
VSD present
Treatment: Fontan/Glenn procedures
= conduit from IVC/SVC to PA

Ebstein's anomaly

Apical displacement of TV leaflets (usually septal TVL)
Atrialization of RV → large RA/small RV
Diagnosis: septal TVL attaches to IVS > 8 mm/m^2 below ant MVL
    AMVL – LV apex/STVL – RV apex > 1.8
Associated with TR/ASD

Pulmonary valve

Uni-/bi-/quadricuspid valve → PS
Congenital absence of PV
Fallot's tetralogy: PS

Ventricular defects

Univentricle

Two atria → one ventricle
Second ventricle hypoplastic/absent

TOE assessment

(1) Accessory chamber
    Hypoplastic or absent
(2) Atrio-ventricular valve function
    2 AV valves 65%
    1 AV valve 35%
(3) Great vessel orientation
    Aorta or PA may arise from either
    Hypoplastic or functioning ventricle
    Associated with TGA
(4) RVOT/LVOT obstruction
    Hypoplastic PA common
(5) Univentricle function
    Response to volume/pressure overload
(6) Venous return
    Associated with TAPVD

Treatment

Aorto-pulmonary shunt:
    Waterson = asc. aorta → PA
    Potts = desc. aorta → LPA
Blalock–Taussig shunt:
    R subclavian artery → RPA
Septation:
    creation of artificial IVS

Great vessels

Fallot's tetralogy

(1) PS: usually infundibular with PA hypoplasia
(2) VSD: perimembranous
(3) Overriding aorta
(4) Concentric RV hypertrophy

Associated with
    Abnormal coronary anatomy (2–5%)
    Secundum ASD
    PDA
    Right-sided aortic arch

Treatment

(1) Unobstructed PV:
    valvulotomy
(2) Two-stage:
    initial aorto-pulmonary shunt
    later valved conduit from RV to PA (Rastelli)

Transposition of great arteries (TGA)

Aorta from RV/PA from LV
Associated with
    VSD
    Secundum ASD
    Abnormal atrio-ventricular (A–V) valves
    LVOT/RVOT obstruction
    PDA
    Abnormal coronary anatomy

Treatment

Early arterial switch procedure
Palliative balloon atrial septostomy with later repair (Mustard)

Truncus arteriosus (TA)

Single trunk from heart provides aorta/PA/coronary arteries
Associated with
    Large VSD
    Abnormal truncal valve

Right-sided aortic arch
Abnormal coronary anatomy

Treatment

Close VSD
Repair/replace truncal valve
Conduit from RV to PA

Patent ductus arteriosus (PDA)

Normal in fetus/closes by third day after birth
Causes L → R shunt with ↑PA flow
Abnormal diastolic flow in PA seen with TOE

Coarctation

Localized defect of media with eccentric narrowing of lumen
Adult type = postductal narrowing
Infantile type = preductal coarctation

Venous return

Total anomalous pulmonary venous drainage (TAPVD)

(1) Supracardiac: PVs → SVC/innominate vein
(2) Cardiac: PVs → RA/coronary sinus
(3) Infracardiac: PVs → IVC/portal vein
(4) Mixed

ASD

Primum ASD

20% of ASDs
Due to incomplete fusion of septum primum
Low in septum (Fig. 8.1)

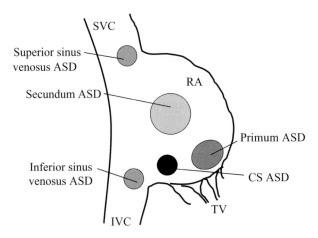

Fig. 8.1

Secundum ASD

70% of ASDs
Due to incomplete development of septum secundum
In region of fossa ovalis (Fig. 8.1)

Patent foramen ovale (PFO)

Present in ~ 25% of population
Incomplete closure of foramen ovale at birth

Sinus venosus ASD

6–8% of ASDs
Superior sinus venosus: high in septum by SVC
Inferior sinus venosus: low in septum by IVC
Associated with TAPVD (Fig. 8.1)

Coronary sinus (CS) ASD

At site of origin of CS (Fig. 8.1)
Associated with unroofed CS/persistent left SVC

Endocardial cushion defects

Due to A–V canal defects

Complete
Large primum ASD
Inlet of IVS deficient with large VSD

Partial
Primum ASD
Cleft MV

VSD

Supracristal

Above level of crista supraventricularis (Fig. 8.2)
Immediately inferior to PV and AV (LCC and RCC)
= infundibular VSD

Infracristal

Inferior and posterior to crista supraventricularis (Fig. 8.2)

(1) Membranous: beneath AV (RCC/NCC)
(2) Muscular: occur post-MI
(3) Inlet VSD

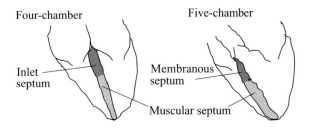

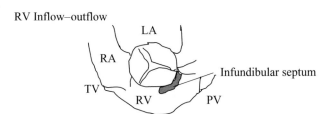

Fig. 8.2

Multiple choice questions

1. The following statements regarding the bicuspid aortic valve are all true except
   A it is associated with ascending aortic aneurysm
   B it is a common site for bacterial endocarditis
   C it occurs in approximately 1–2% of the population
   D aortic incompetence does not occur
   E it is associated with coarctation of the aorta
2. In Ebstein's anomaly
   A there is apical displacement of the mitral valve leaflets
   B diagnosis is made when the septal tricuspid valve leaflet attaches to the interventricular septum more than 8 mm above the anterior mitral valve leaflet
   C tricuspid regurgitation is not a feature
   D there is an association with atrial septal defect
   E atrialisation of the left ventricle occurs

3. Regarding congenital ventricular defects,
   A the accessory chamber is usually hypertrophied
   B there is an association with total anomalous pulmonary venous drainage
   C two atrioventricular valves occur in 35% of cases
   D echocardiographic assessment of the right ventricular outflow tract is not important
   E it can be treated by the Rastelli procedure

4. Fallot's tetralogy
   A includes a muscular ventricular septal defect
   B has abnormal coronary anatomy in 50% of cases
   C is treated by the Mustard procedure
   D usually includes eccentric right ventricular hypertrophy
   E can be initially managed with an aorto-pulmonary shunt

5. The following statements regarding congenital heart defects are all true except
   A transposition of the great arteries is associated with secundum atrial septal defect
   B truncus arteriosus is associated with abnormal coronary anatomy
   C patent ductus arteriosus causes a right to left shunt
   D adult type coarctation involves postductal narrowing
   E in total anomalous pulmonary venous drainage, pulmonary veins may drain into the coronary sinus

6. Regarding atrial septal defects (ASDs)
   A 70% are primum ASDs
   B 20% are secundum ASDs
   C 17% are sinus venosus ASDs
   D secundum ASDs occur low in the interatrial septum
   E primum ASDs are due to incomplete fusion of the septum primum

7. Endocardial cushion defects (ECDs)
   A involve aortic valve defects
   B in complete ECDs there is usually a small ventricular septal defect
   C partial ECDs are associated with cleft mitral valve
   D complete ECDs have a small secundum atrial septal defect
   E partial ECDs have a large secundum atrial septal defect

8. Regarding ventricular septal defects (VSDs)

    A supracristal VSDs include membranous VSDs

    B membranous VSDs usually occur beneath the right and non-coronary cusps of the aortic valve

    C infracristal VSDs include infundibular VSDs

    D infracristal VSDs do not occur post-myocardial infarction

    E infundibular VSDs are best seen on a mid-oesophageal four-chamber view

9

Extracardiac anatomy

Pericardium

Effusion

Normal pericardial sac contains 20–30 ml of fluid from subepicardial lymphatics

Causes
(1) Idiopathic
(2) Cardiac: CCF, post-MI, post-cardiac surgery
(3) Metabolic: hypoalbuminaemia, uraemia, hypothyroidism
(4) Infective: bacterial, TB, viral, fungal
(5) Trauma
(6) Connective tissue disease: SLE, rheumatoid arthritis
(7) Neoplasm
(8) Drugs: hydralazine
(9) Radiotherapy

Size
(1) Small: < 100 ml
     localized behind posterior LV
(2) Moderate: 100–500 ml
(3) Large: > 500 ml
     swinging of heart in fluid
     electrical alternans on ECG
Chronic effusion causes fibrinous exudates on pericardial surface
Fibrin strands appear as 'soap-suds' on visceral pericardium

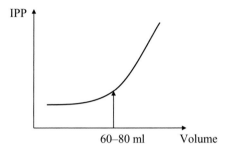

Fig. 9.1

Tamponade

Impairment of diastolic filling caused by raised intrapericardial
pressure (IPP)
Due to

(1) rapid accumulation of small amount of fluid
(2) gradual collection of large volume of fluid

IPP dependent on compliance of pericardium and volume within
　　pericardium
As intra-pericardial volume increases, IPP increases (Fig. 9.1)
As IPP↑ cardiac volume is maintained by increasing venous pressure to
　　maintain venous return
When IPP = venous pressure (volume ~ 60–80 ml) → steep part of
　　compliance curve
When IPP > venous pressure → stroke volume falls
RV filling pressure = LV filling pressure

Effect of respiration
(1) Normal

　　　Inspiration　→ Fall in intrapleural pressure
　　　　　　　　→ This fall transmitted to IPP
　　　　　　　　→ Expansion of RA and RV into pericardial space
　　　　　　　　→ ↑Venous return to right side

(2) Tamponade

> Inspiration $\rightarrow$ Fall in IPP less than normal
> $\rightarrow$ RV fills
> $\rightarrow$ RV unable to expand into pericardial space
> $\rightarrow$ RV expands to the left
> $\rightarrow$ IVS shifts to the left
> $\rightarrow$ LV filling compromised
> $\rightarrow$ $\downarrow$LVEDV
> $\rightarrow$ $\downarrow$CO and $\downarrow$SBP during inspiration

Onset of systole: $\downarrow$RAP = 'x' descent
Onset of diastole: no fall in RAP = no 'y' descent
Right-sided filling becomes monophasic (confined to systole)
Transient pressure gradient reversal: IPP > RAP/RVP
$\rightarrow$ RV wall inversion in diastole
$\rightarrow$ RA wall inversion in late diastole/early systole
$\uparrow$venous return to right side $\rightarrow$ $\uparrow$RV volume
$\rightarrow$ LV compromise
$\rightarrow$ $\uparrow$TTF by 80%/$\downarrow$TMF by 40%

Pericarditis

Pericardium becomes rigid due to
  Inflammation
  Fibrosis
  Calcification
  Neoplasms
Impedes diastolic filling

Causes
(1) Hereditary
(2) Metabolic: uraemia
(3) Infection: bacterial, viral, parasitic
(4) Trauma
(5) Connective tissue disease: polyarteritis nodosa, SLE

Table 9.1 Constrictive vs. restrictive pathophysiology

Constrictive	Restrictive
Thickened calcified pericardium	Normal pericardium
Pulsus paradoxus	
Normal PA pressures	↑PA pressures
MAPSE preserved	MAPSE reduced
Large respiratory variation in TTF and TMF	Minimal (<5%) respiratory
Inspiration → ↑TTF/↓TMF	variation in TTF and TMF
Respiratory variation in pulmonary venous flow	
Inspiration → ↑RVSP/↓LVSP	Inspiration → ↓RVSP/↓LVSP
Hepatic vein flow → ↓D/↑DR	Hepatic vein flow → ↑SR

(6) Neoplasms

(7) Post-cardiac surgery

(8) Radiotherapy

Diagnosis:

    normal ventricular size

    ↓diastolic function

    IVC/HV dilated

    pericardial thickening

Early rapid ventricular filling (rapid 'y' descent), which stops abruptly as limit of ventricular expansion achieved

Respiratory variations in intrapleural pressure not transmitted to heart due to dense pericardial encasement

Constrictive vs. restrictive physiology (Table 9.1)

Limitation to diastolic ventricular filling occurs earlier in CONSTRICTIVE pathology because of fixed volume within the pericardial sac

Myocardial relaxation prolonged in RESTRICTIVE disease

Variation of IVRT on inspiration with CONSTRICTIVE pathology

Aortic disease

Atherosclerosis

Severe disease of descending aorta increases likelihood of aortic arch disease

Grading

I: Minimal intimal thickening
II: Extensive, widespread intimal thickening
III: Sessile atheroma
IV: Atheroma protruding into aortic lumen
V: Mobile, protruding atheroma

Aneurysm

Dilatation of all layers of aortic wall

Causes

Atherosclerosis
Cystic medial necrosis
Trauma
Congenital (Marfan's)
Syphilis

Affects ascending aorta/aortic arch/thoracic and abdominal aorta

Dissection

Degeneration/destruction of media
Associated with

Hypertension
Connective tissue disease
Turner's syndrome
Coarctation

Table 9.2 Comparison of Stanford type A and B dissection

	Stanford A	Stanford B
Frequency (%)	70	30
Age	50	70
Male : female	2:1	3:1
Associated ↑BP (%)	50	80
AI (%)	50	10
Acute mortality (%)	90	40

Classification

(1) Stanford (Table 9.2)

   A: proximal tear

   B: distal tear

(2) De Bakey

   I: proximal tear, extending distally

   II: proximal tear

   IIIA: distal tear, extending proximally

   IIIB: distal tear

Management

Stanford A → surgery

Stanford B → medical therapy

Multiple choice questions

1. Causes of pericardial effusion include all of the following except

   A Wilson's disease

   B neoplastic disease

   C trauma

D rheumatoid arthritis

E radiotherapy

2. **Regarding intrapericardial pressure (IPP)**

   A when IPP increases to equal venous pressure, right ventricular filling pressure will equal left ventricular filling pressure

   B IPP is independent of intrapericardial volume

   C when IPP exceeds venous pressure stroke volume increases

   D IPP equals venous pressure at a volume of 500 ml

   E IPP is independent of pericardial compliance

3. **In adults, cardiac tamponade**

   A is caused by an intrapericardial volume of 20 ml

   B is due to a gradual accumulation of a small amount of fluid

   C causes a rapid 'y' descent on the central venous waveform

   D causes right atrial wall eversion in diastole

   E causes right ventricular wall inversion in diastole

4. **The following statements about pericarditis are all true except**

   A it is caused by systemic lupus erythematosus

   B late ventricular filling occurs due to high intraventricular pressure

   C it impedes diastolic filling

   D respiratory variations in intrapleural pressure are not transmitted to the heart

   E the hepatic vein is usually dilated

5. **In constrictive cardiac pathology**

   A mitral annular plane systolic excursion is reduced

   B pulmonary hypertension is common

   C right ventricular systolic pressure decreases on inspiration

   D left ventricular systolic pressure decreases on inspiration

   E transmitral flow increases on inspiration

6. **In restrictive cardiac pathology**

   A the pericardium appears thickened and calcified

   B left ventricular systolic pressure decreases on inspiration

   C pulsus paradoxus is a feature

   D isovolumic relaxation time varies on inspiration

   E there is increased respiratory variation in pulmonary venous flow

7. All of the following may cause thoracic aortic aneurysm except
   A cystic medial necrosis
   B syphilis
   C gonorrhoea
   D Marfan's syndrome
   E atherosclerosis
8. The following statements about thoracic aortic dissection are all true except
   A it is associated with coarctation of the aorta
   B Stanford type A has a higher acute mortality than type B
   C De Bakey type II involves a proximal aortic dissection
   D surgery is indicated in Stanford type A
   E aortic valve incompetence is more common in Stanford type B than type A

10

Haemodynamic calculations

Doppler equation

$$\text{velocity} = cf_D/2\,f_O\,\cos\theta$$
$$f_D = 2vf_O\,\cos\theta/c$$

Bernoulli equation

$$P_1 - P_2 = \left[1/2\rho\left(V_2^2 - V_1^2\right)\right] + [\rho^2\,dV/dt.ds] + [RV^2]$$

Convective	Flow	Viscous
acceleration	acceleration	friction

Modified Bernoulli $\Delta P = 4V^2$

Intracardiac pressures

$$\text{RVSP} = \text{RAP} + 4V^2 \; (\text{TR})$$
$$\text{PADP} = \text{RAP} + 4V^2 \; (\text{PI})$$
$$\text{LAP} = \text{SBP} - 4V^2 \; (\text{MR})$$
$$\text{LVEDP} = \text{DBP} - 4V^2 \; (\text{AI})$$

Flow

$$\text{Flow} = \text{Area} \times \text{Velocity}$$
$$\text{SV} = \text{Area} \times \text{VTI}$$

Aortic valve

Aortic stenosis

$$\Delta P = 4V^2$$
$$\text{AVA} = \text{Area}_{\text{LVOT}} \times V_{\text{max}_{\text{LVOT}}} / V_{\text{max}_{\text{AV}}}$$
$$\text{AVA} = \text{SV}_{\text{AV}} / \text{VTI}_{\text{AV}}$$

Aortic incompetence

$$\text{RF\%} = \text{SV}_{\text{LVOT}} - \text{SV}_{\text{MV}} / \text{SV}_{\text{LVOT}}$$

Mitral valve

Mitral stenosis

$$\Delta P = 4V^2$$
$$\text{MVA} = 220/\text{PHT}$$
$$\text{MVA} = \text{Area}_{\text{LVOT}} \times \text{VTI}_{\text{LVOT}} / \text{VTI}_{\text{MV}}$$
$$\text{MVA} = 6.28r^2 \times \alpha / 180 \times V_{\text{alias}} / V_{\text{max}_{\text{MV}}}$$

Mitral regurgitation

$$\text{RV} = (\text{Area}_{\text{MV}} \times \text{VTI}_{\text{MV}}) - (\text{Area}_{\text{LVOT}} \times \text{VTI}_{\text{LVOT}})$$
$$\text{RF} = \text{SV}_{\text{MV}} - \text{SV}_{\text{LVOT}} / \text{SV}_{\text{MV}}$$
$$\text{ERO} = 6.28r^2 \times V_{\text{alias}} / V_{\text{max}_{\text{MR}}}$$

Multiple choice questions

1. A peak Doppler velocity of 4 m/s across the aortic valve equates to a peak pressure gradient of
   A 4 mmHg
   B 16 mmHg
   C 32 mmHg
   D 64 mmHg
   E 80 mmHg

The following data apply to Questions 2–4
   Right atrial pressure = 10 mmHg
   Left ventricular end diastolic/left atrial pressure = 18 mmHg
   Tricuspid regurgitation jet peak velocity = 3 m/s
   Mitral regurgitation jet peak velocity = 5 m/s
   Pulmonary insufficiency jet peak velocity = 1 m/s
   Aortic incompetence jet peak velocity = 4 m/s
   Mean arterial pressure = 94 mmHg

2. The right ventricular systolic pressure is
   A 46 mmHg
   B 36 mmHg
   C 26 mmHg
   D 16 mmHg
   E 12 mmHg

3. The systemic systolic pressure is
   A 82 mmHg
   B 100 mmHg
   C 118 mmHg
   D 130 mmHg
   E 146 mmHg

4. The systemic diastolic pressure is
   A 56 mmHg
   B 64 mmHg
   C 72 mmHg
   D 82 mmHg
   E 88 mmHg

The following data apply to Questions 5–6

    Left ventricular outflow tract area $= 3$ cm^2

    Left ventricular maximum velocity $= 1.5$ m/s

    Aortic valve maximum velocity $= 4.5$ m/s

    Aortic valve VTI $= 40$ cm

5. Aortic valve area is

  A 0.5 cm^2

  B 1.0 cm^2

  C 1.2 cm^2

  D 1.5 cm^2

  E 2.0 cm^2

6. Aortic valve stroke volume is

  A 40 ml

  B 50 ml

  C 60 ml

  D 70 ml

  E 80 ml

The following data apply to Questions 7–8

    Mitral valve area $= 5$ cm^2

    Mitral valve VTI $= 16$ cm

    Mitral regurgitation jet peak velocity $= 4$ m/s

    Left ventricular outflow tract stroke volume $= 50$ ml

7. Mitral valve regurgitant volume is

  A 14 ml

  B 24 ml

  C 30 ml

  D 38 ml

  E 50 ml

8. Mitral valve regurgitant fraction is approximately

  A 25%

  B 38%

  C 48%

  D 60%

  E 80%

MCQ answers

Chapter 1

1. C	8. E	15. D
2. B	9. A	16. A
3. D	10. C	17. D
4. B	11. C	18. E
5. B	12. A	19. C
6. A	13. A	20. C
7. D	14. E	

Chapter 2

1. E	3. E
2. A	4. C

Chapter 3

1. E	7. B	13. B
2. C	8. C	14. B
3. C	9. D	15. A
4. D	10. E	16. D
5. B	11. E	
6. A	12. C	

Chapter 4

1. D	5. E	9. D
2. C	6. C	10. B
3. A	7. E	11. A
4. E	8. D	12. C

Chapter 5

1. E	3. C
2. A	4. B

Chapter 6

1. A	5. E	9. B
2. A	6. C	10. A
3. B	7. D	11. D
4. B	8. C	12. A

Chapter 7

1. D	3. B
2. D	4. D

Chapter 8

1. D	5. C
2. D	6. E
3. B	7. C
4. E	8. B

Chapter 9

1. A	5. D
2. A	6. B
3. E	7. C
4. B	8. E

Chapter 10

1. D	5. B
2. A	6. A
3. C	7. C
4. D	8. B

References

Curry, T. S., Dowdy, J. E., & Murry, R. C. (eds.). *Christensen's Physics of Diagnostic Radiology*, 4th edn. Philadelphia: Lea & Febiger, 1990.

Feigenbaum, H. (ed.). *Echocardiography*, 5th edn. Philadelphia: Lea & Febiger, 1993.

Kahn, R. A., Konstadt, S. N., Louie, E. K., Aronson, S., & Thys, D. M. In Kaplan, J. A. (ed). *Cardiac Anesthesia*, 4th edn. Philadelphia: W. B. Saunders Co., 1999.

Kawahara, T., Yamagishi, M., Seo, H. *et al.* Application of Doppler color flow imaging to determine valve area in mitral stenosis. *J. Am. Coll. Cardiol.* 1991; **18**: 85–92.

Martin, K. In Hoskins, P. R., Thrush, A., Martin, K., & Whittingham, T. A. (eds.). *Diagnostic Ultrasound Physics and Equipment*. London: Greenwich Medical Media Ltd, 2003.

Peters, P. J. & Reinhardt, S. The echocardiographic evaluation of intracardiac masses: a review. *J. Am. Soc. Echocardiogr.* 2006; **19**: 230–40.

Practice Guidelines for Perioperative Transesophageal Echocardiography: A report by the American Society of Anesthesiologists and the Society of Cardiovascular Anesthesiologists Task Force on perioperative transesophageal echocardiography. *Anesthesiology* 1996; **84**: 986–1006.

Rafferty, T. D. (ed.). *Basics of Transesophageal Echocardiography*. Philadelphia: Churchill Livingstone, 1995.

Reisner, S. A. & Meltzer, R. S. Normal values of prosthetic valve Doppler echocardiographic parameters: a review. *J. Am. Soc. Echocardiogr.* 1988; **1**: 201–10.

Ribakove, G. H., Katz, E. S., Ealloway, A. C. *et al.* Surgical implications of transesophageal echocardiography to grade the atheromatous aortic arch. *Ann. Thorac. Surg.* 1992; **53**: 758–61.

Rodriguez, L., Thomas, J. D., Monterroso, V. *et al.* Validation of the proximal flow convergence method. Calculation of orifice area in patients with mitral stenosis. *Circulation* 1993; **88**: 1157–65.

Shanewise, J. S., Cheung, A. T., Aronson, S. *et al.* ASE/SCA guidelines for performing a comprehensive intraoperative multiplane transesophageal echocardiogram examination: recommendations of the American Society of Echocardiography Council for intraoperative echocardiography and the Society of Cardiovascular Anesthesiologists Task Force for certification in perioperative transesophageal echocardiography. *Anesth. Analg.* 1999; **89**: 870–84.

Wallace, L. In *Annual Comprehensive Review and TEE Update: Clinical Decision Making in the Cardiac Surgery Patient*, 2003.

Weyman, A. E. (ed.). *Principles and Practice of Echocardiography*, 2nd edn. Philadelphia: Lea & Febiger, 1994.

Index

Note: page numbers in *italics* refer to tables